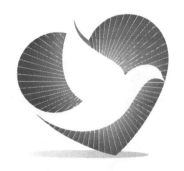

BIBLICAL PRESCRIPTIONS for LIFE™

Rosemarie Briggs

Small Group Study Guide

Printed in the United States of America

Second Printing, 2016

ISBN 9780997160000

Heartwise Ministries

8831 Forest Creek Lane, Ooltewah, TN 37363

biblicalprescriptionsforlife.com

heartwiseministries.org

THIS STUDY IS DEDICATED to an unforgettable young lady who prayed without words we could understand, but who demonstrated an authentic life with God that spoke volumes. Kala loved to talk to God and she wanted people to pray with her and for her.

Kala is still teaching us that God uses everything for our good and that when we worship, we see God. And that as we behold God, we are healed.

Kala Akins
February 15, 1990 – December 17, 2015

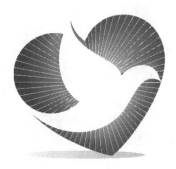

CONTENTS

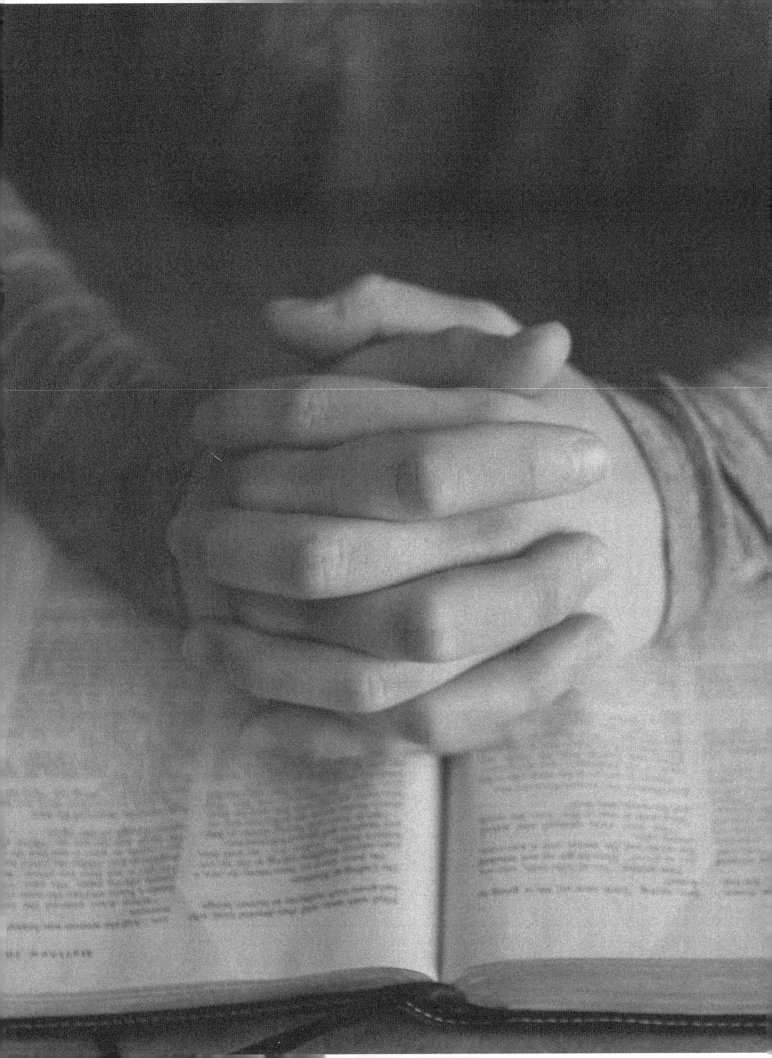

PROLOGUE

This study may launch you on one of the most significant journeys you've ever made. It's the path out of the ordinary, go-with-the-flow, hurried and harried quagmire of living, to a growing, thriving, higher quality of life. If you're ready for a change then you're ready for this study. Ideally, you've found a small group of other people who are just as eager to start this journey with you.

This study was written to improve health and serve as another approach to spread the gospel. Christ met the needs of others and introduced them to the Father for ultimate healing. The study is intended to help your physician in your care. Please make your doctor aware of the changes you are making. This might enable your physician to change your medication regimen. The physicians I work with welcome new ways to help their patients. In the office, often we just do not have the time to educate and develop practical steps to combat the complexities of chronic disease. The study will also help to prevent the health problems that are now so prevalent in our society. The practical steps you will learn and incorporate will treat will treat the entire body in the context of our integrated, amazing design. This is termed wholism.

If you are leading, review the leader guide material at biblicalprescriptionsforlife.com/leader for suggestions to help your study. Be flexible. Some may want to move slower and spread the study over more time. Some may choose to spend more or less time on the study each day. This is up to you. The study was designed with a format and length similar to other Bible studies. It is perfectly acceptable to have fun during our journey together.

Here are some very important things to consider—so important that we've put them here before you even get started.

1. **This course is simple, success-oriented, and sustainable.** The material is clear. The action steps are simple, success-oriented, scalable, and sustainable. You start where you are and end up where you want be be—living a healing lifestyle. We try to make changes one step at a time.

2. **The wellness plan in this study is not intended to replace the counsel of your primary care physician.** We encourage you to consult with a medical professional familiar with you before you begin any of the changes suggested in this course.

3. **You'll get more from this study if you do the work in the context of a community with regular time scheduled for face-to-face, life-on-life connection.** We were created for relationship and, as we'll learn later, relationship is a central component to whole-life wellness.

4. **You will get more from this study if you actually follow the plan.** Trust us, it's not overwhelming. In fact, more than 9 out of every 10 people who have completed this course have told us that they cannot imagine living any other way. They've discovered a wellness lifestyle they can actually live with!

5. **You will not be judged.** Success is taking the journey from wherever you start. We will stay positive as we move forward.

6. **Life is about direction, not perfection.** None of us will achieve perfection in this life. Striving for it creates its own set of pathologies—relationally and physiologically. Don't beat yourself up or set an unachievable goal. Instead, start *moving toward* whole-life wellness.

7. **You will experience lifelong transformation.** Whether you can barely walk across the room today or are training for your first 10k, you'll find clear, simple, and sustainable changes you can make right away to transform your wellness level; probably even transform your life.

I've written *Biblical Prescriptions for Life* using the Bible as the source of truth. To get the most from this study, we must agree on two very important things before we go any farther:

1. **If we're serious about learning from God and making sustainable change in our lives, we need to dig deep into what He's told us.** I want you to start reading with a purpose. One of the best ways for doing this is to mark key words from the Bible passages we'll examine and record everything you learn from them as you read. I want you to search through the Bible like you're looking for the clues for the whole-life healing God longs for us to discover. You will discover Biblical Prescriptions that will transform your health.

2. **I want you to realize—to believe—that you're hearing from a real person when you listen to God through His Word.** God is actually Three in One: the Father, the Son and the Holy Spirit. The Holy Spirit opens our *understanding* to the Word of God. The Father *redeems* us through the perfect, *sacrificial* work of His Son Jesus. God is the Divine Trinity and He desires to enjoy a relationship with each and every one of us.

    Before you begin your time studying *Biblical Prescriptions for Life* each day, ask God to lead you into all truth. You might pray like this: *"Father—thank you for wanting to speak to me today. I want to learn what you say about my health and relationship with you. Thank you Jesus, for making our relationship possible. And thank you, Holy Spirit for promising to lead me into all truth. Amen."*

In writing this study, I have leaned on the experience I have gained over the years practicing medicine. Many other physicians, teachers, patients and friends have contributed to this study. Their input has been invaluable. I have tried to place a daunting amount of material into a framework that is practical based on experiences of others and myself. This has been challenging, as we want a program that is not too complicated, is doable, economical, and just makes sense. This study is about turning to God for your healthcare concerns. We pray that God uses us to help others in a practical way. Change must happen for the right reasons.

Are you ready? You're probably more ready than you realize! Thousands of others have begun to experience a new path to lifelong, whole-life wellness that's definitely more doable than you've ever expected. Let's start the journey, moving one step at a time.

—James Marcum, MD

My Biblical Prescriptions for Life

Use this page to keep a running list of the Biblical Prescriptions for Life you are adding into your new healthy lifestyle. As you complete each week of study, transfer the Biblical Prescriptions you plan to keep using to this list as your at-a-glance chart.

I commit to	My Biblical Prescription for Life	Day 1	2	3	4	5	6	7

My Small Group Relationships

Life is meant to be lived in relationship. God designed us to heal in community. Use this chart to keep your Biblical Prescriptions for Life small group at the front of your mind.

Name	The Best Way I Can Care for Them	Mobile Number

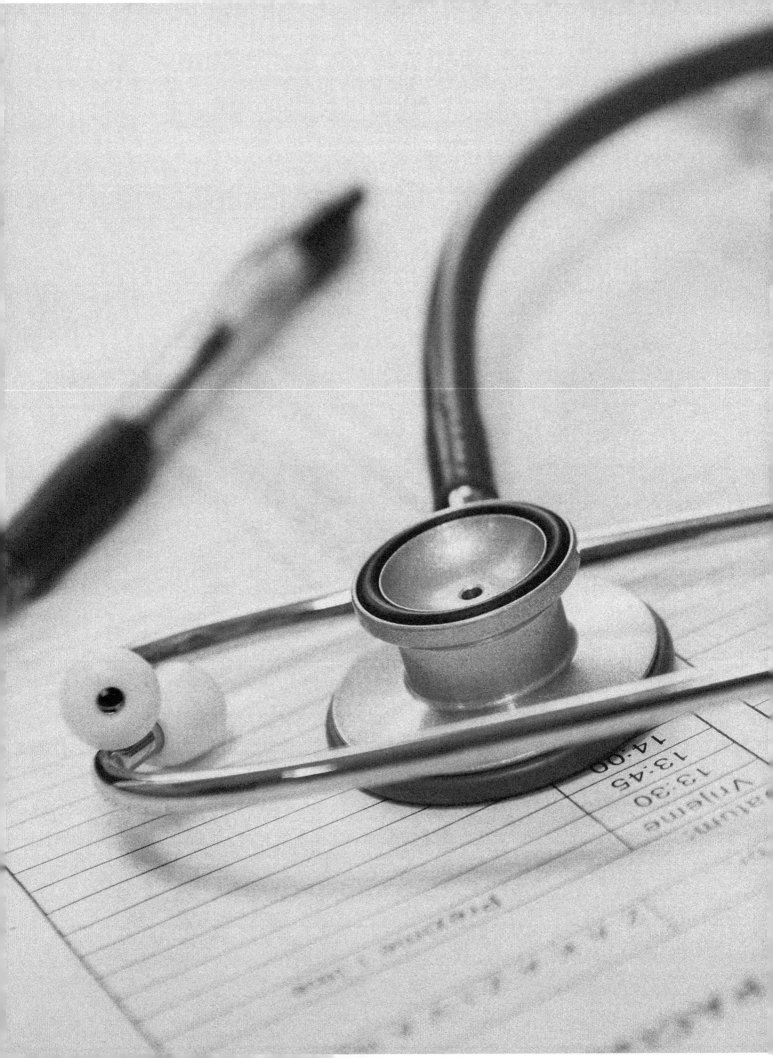

WEEK 1

"The Doctor Will Be Right with You."

Michelle was 40 years old when she walked into my cardiology exam room. She had invested 20 years of her life as a legal assistant at a prestigious downtown law practice. Unfortunately, things were not going well for her.

At the law firm, she wore high heels everyday—part of the corporate dress code. After two decades of this, she started having foot pain. When she couldn't bear it any longer, she made an appointment with a podiatrist. He found a problem in her calcaneus (heel bone) that required surgery.

After the operation, Michelle had to wear a boot while her foot healed. Because of this, she stopped exercising and started gaining weight. Months went by. She visited her primary care physician concerned about her constant thirst and increasingly frequent trips to the bathroom. You guessed it: her doctor diagnosed type 2 diabetes and put her on the drug Metformin.

Metformin made her hungry. So Michelle ate lots of salty foods. Before long her blood pressure soared. Her doctor sent her to a blood pressure specialist who immediately put her on Norvasc.

Norvasc caused her to retain water and her legs swelled so her doctors prescribed a fluid pill. This drug pulled potassium and magnesium out of her body so they added supplements to keep her electrolytes replenished.

As you can imagine, Michelle was getting discouraged and wasn't sleeping well at night. She started experiencing acid reflux and her doctors suggested an acid-blocking medicine. When she still didn't sleep well, they gave her a sleeping pill.

In spite of all this, Michelle still had pain in her foot.

By this time, because she was heavier, less agile, and dealing with chronic pain, she no longer fit the "standard" at work. She wasn't the ideal they wanted. So after 20 years with the legal firm, they let her go. As you and I can relate, this was quite a blow to her emotionally. So her doctor referred her to a psychiatrist who started her on an anti-depressant.

Since her foot still wasn't healing correctly, her doctors sent Michelle—remember, she's only 40 years young—to a pain clinic where she was introduced to a narcotic called Lortab. Unfortunately, the Lortab caused her bowels to slow down and Michelle felt bloated. Then her bowels backed up and she contracted an infection of the intestines called diverticulitis and was given an antibiotic. The antibiotic changed the bacteria in the bowel. Another infection, C-difficile-colitis developed. Next her doctors started her on another antibiotic called Flagyl.

Michelle was seeing an infectious disease specialist, a podiatrist, a psychiatrist, an internist, and a blood pressure specialist. She came to my cardiology practice because she now was experiencing chest pain. All the doctors were trying to help Michelle, but one stressor led to another.

Whew!

I told Michelle, if we can understand the underlying cause of a problem, we could better find successful treatments. Sometimes in life, there's stress we can control. Sometimes there's stress we can't control. And oftentimes, there's stress we don't even know about. But no matter the cause, the chemistry of stress can snowball. And it may lead to more symptoms! Just ask Michelle (who is now doing much better). Michelle asked me to tell her story. To treat Michelle, I needed to know more than the symptoms. I needed to understand the cause and the stressors involved.

I'll bring us back to Michelle a little later.

VIDEO GUIDE 1

How's Life Working for You?

VIDEO (20 minutes)

Major Bible verses:

- Psalm 46:10
- Matthew 11:28

Who is Michelle? What stands out in your mind about her? Is there anything in her life to which you can relate?

Age _____

Symptoms _____

Lifestyle _____

Relationships _____

How do you define stress?

What is Dr. Marcum's definition of stress?

Identify at least three stressors in your life.

1.

2

3.

Are you currently having symptoms?

The human brain is an amazing, masterfully designed organ with three main functional areas. What are the three functional layers?

1. _____
2. _____
3. _____

What are the functions of the layers?

Area 1: _____
Area 2: _____
Area 3: _____

How do the different layers affect your life?

_____

Under stress, the brain seeks functions to remain safe. When under stress the brain_____. From the ideas you heard in the video, what are some ways you can make purposeful changes when under stress? To move functions to the third layer of the brain is termed _____.

Our *Biblical Prescriptions for Life* for Week 1

1. _____
2. _____
3. _____

Group Discussion (20 Minutes)
While watching the video, what most impacted you? Why?

_____

Like Michelle, are you ready to get real? If so, you and your group might find this is the perfect time to share your personal answers to the big question—"*How are you doing*?" Along with the members of your group, each of you finish this sentence—"*I want to change*_____"

LIVING IN COMMUNITY

We were created to live in real, meaningful relationships: bearing one another's burdens, and sharing joys, and sorrows. When we live to give, we receive more than we give.

Take a moment right after today's meeting and connect with at least one other person—or if your group is less than 7 people, try to connect with each person and exchange mobile numbers or email addresses. Then call each other during the week to encourage one another in practicing what you're learning *together*, in community.

Name	The Best Way I Can Care for Them	Mobile Number

INDIVIDUAL REFLECTION

As we listened to each other, what was your top-level take-away thought from this week's time together? (This is just for you. Write it here.) _____

BEING MISSIONAL

Is there someone you know outside of this group who might be encouraged and excited to learn what God can do through small, simple, sustainable changes? It's not too late to invite them to join your group for Session 2 next week. Write their name here and plan how you'll contact them.

_____

_____

_____

COMMITMENT

This week, I am going to DO at least one of the following simple Biblical Prescriptions for Life:

I commit to	Biblical Prescriptions for Life	Day 1	2	3	4	5	6	7
	Read aloud 5x each day. Practice, memorize & recite:							
	Matthew 11:28 "Come to me all who labor and are heavy laden, and I will give you rest. Take my yoke upon you, and learn from me, for I am gentle and lowly in heart, and you will find rest for your souls."							
	Psalm 46:10 "Be still and know that I am God. I will be exalted among the nations. I will be exalted in the earth!"							

If you missed a session or want to review one, go to biblicalprescriptionsforlife.com to stream Dr. Marcum's audio and video

WEEK 1

Even if Today is the Worst Day, it's The First Day of the Rest of Your Life

It was the most sobering day of my life. It made me call my education, my training—even my *life calling*—into question.

You could say healthcare is in my DNA. My father was an anesthetist. A gentle, generous and wise man, he demonstrated a life of commitment to helping others. He showed me the most rewarding path was the journey of lifelong learning and serving. He's my hero to this day.

I followed my father into the medical field, earning my medical degree from the University of Texas at San Antonio and completing my internship and residency in internal medicine at the Medical Center of Delaware. I fulfilled my fellowship in cardiovascular disease at the University of Kentucky at Lexington and then committed my education and resources to becoming the best cardiologist I could be.

I was now in my second year of residency as a member of a prestigious internal medicine residency program in Wilmington, Delaware. It was the fall of 1992 and I was on the edge of a case that would shape the rest of my life.

"Tom" was a 32-years-young man who came to the hospital with a malignancy. The medical team in charge of his care thought that a bone marrow transplant was the way to go. So we began treating him with a powerful chemotherapy to kill the malignant cells. As is usually the case with such procedures, this treatment also killed many of his good cells as well.

I remember observing his white and red blood cell count drop as his bone marrow succumbed to the treatment. We had to give frequent transfusions and then give him various antibiotics at the slightest sign of infection. Tom suffered greatly under this treatment, both physically and emotionally. Tom was a strong fire fighter. He was in a new and for-eign world. The medications made him ill; he was nauseated most of the time. He lost his appetite and had to receive nutrition through the veins. He lost his hair. His once strong body became weak and frail. My patient was courageous even though he was isolated in a sterile room and could see his family for only limited periods of time.

Soon, it was time for the bone marrow transplant. Hopes ran high that the malignancy was gone. Yes, he was gaining strength, but the strain on his system, all the stress, had left him looking much older than thirty-two. While I was amazed at the science and technology surrounding the case, deep down I felt something was missing. Our hopes, the patient's hopes and his family's hopes were all tied into what modern medicine could do—and I was part of that.

Not long after the marrow transplant, my patient Tom became desperately ill. A sudden infection gripped his body in a terrible embrace. Despite the use of ventilators, dialysis, and intravenous medications, he died. As he was nearing the end, I was in his room, caring for him. I remember him looking at me with unspoken questions in his eyes, but he passed away before I could provide the answers. This bothered me a great deal. Everything I knew—everything that modern medicine had to offer—was not enough to save him.

That's when I turned to God with that same, questioning look in my eyes. There had to be more—more information, more insights and more truth than what I'd been taught. Right then and there, I prayed for God to open my eyes, help me find truth and give me the courage to speak out when others were silent.

And so began, a slow journey that continues to this day. I started looking beyond my medical textbooks for answers. Ultimately, I began searching for *healing* truth where most people search for *spiritual* truth—in the pages of God's Holy Word. What I found was astonishing!

In spite of utilizing the world's best medical training, drug therapy and technology, I learned there was more to healing.

As you read, I hope you'll find the answers you need. As you do the lessons, watch the videos and interact with your group members, I hope you'll also discover that there is something more than what you've been taught. That discovery just might change your life forever.

DAY 1

What You Don't Know May Be Killing You

It was very early in my life as a physician that I faced a sobering truth—the best that western medicine had to offer was often not addressing the larger issues. I was treating symptoms, not causes. I knew there must be something more.

Remember the story of Michelle? She was an intelligent 40-year-old in the corporate world who described herself as "falling apart physically, emotionally, relationally" when she first walked into the exam room.

In clinician's terms, she "presented" with chest pain. That means when she arrived to our medical office, the symptom we could see and the one she reported was chest pain. As you think back on her story, you also remember there was a long list of other symptoms and a growing roll call of doctors who were treating them even before she showed up in our waiting room. It had all started with foot pain. Or had it?

Well, yes and no.

Our feet weren't designed to be crammed into a pair of fashionable high heels. When we compress bones and restrict blood flow to muscles and supporting tissue within very complex structures (there are more than 26 individual bones in each human foot!), and then add all our body weight in a position and posture they were never meant to withstand, there's going to be stress. Just the pivoting required to accommodate the high heel on each shoe is enough to cause lower leg injury. Add that to the unnaturally compressed and tightly restricted condition of the feet and you're no longer walking or standing in a way consistent with your design.

A recent University of Alabama study noted that between 2002 and 2012, injuries from high-heeled shoes *doubled*. In that study, there were 123,355 mishaps including 3,294 emergency room visits with 19% of those with broken foot bones. The study author ends the article with these understated words: "It would be worthwhile to understand the risks."

Ladies, I've heard many of you tell me what my wife used to say after a long day on her feet in high heels. "Boy, do my feet hurt" and, "I'm so glad to have those [shoes] off!"

What I meant by "yes and no" is that *yes*, her foot pain was the first symptom that started a snowball that rolled through surgery, multiple prescription drugs, and a long list of specialists. I meant *no*, in the sense that even Michelle's foot pain was not the root cause. Behind her symptoms—and ours—there's something much larger at play. The hidden stressors of life may be causing silent changes in our physiology that may eventually result in a symptom and a trip to the provider.

Consider this formula for pain: Going against our original design > stress > stress chemistry > damage to our bodies > symptoms > eventually, abnormal physiology and/or disease. There is a place for modern medicine. There are times when a patient's stress is acute and doctors need to take advantage of the medicines and technology needed to successfully treat the emergency. The treatment gets us over the hump, however, even in those cases, the treatment often does not address the cause of the problem.

Through *Biblical Prescriptions for Life*, we are going to unpack the *cause behind the symptoms*.

WRAPPING IT UP

Imagine you have scheduled an appointment with my office. Maybe you want to make sure your cardiovascular system is functioning well. Maybe you have a symptom that's causing concern and you've finally made time to get it checked out. Whatever the reason for your appointment, you've made the decision to allow me to become involved in your life.

Well, during this our first week together I want to meet your needs just as I do with each patient who comes to my office. I want to find out what the immediate symptoms are and work backward to find a cause.

The first video provided you and your small group the proper setting for talking frankly about each of your lives and the symptoms you experience. I hope you really opened up with each other during that session. When we're serious about getting healthy, we stop holding back. We become transparent. We become honest. We get real. And we connect to others who are committed to journeying with us in grace and love.

To complete our time together today, I'd like to bring you back to two key components to *Biblical Prescriptions for Life*—Community and Commitment—as we take steps to improve our lives.

LIVING IN COMMUNITY

Plan a time today when you'll stop and contact one of your small group members. You need this as much as they do. I believe you're up to the challenge to overcome the fear of awkwardness, procrastination, and passivity. Call them. Text them. But do it today. Remember, part of our original design is that we were created for relationship in community. This is a very significant component in becoming healthy. Refer to the chart on page 4.

BEING MISSIONAL

What did God show you today in your study? Ask Him to show you a way to start a conversation about what you discovered with someone outside of your group. Talk to your study buddy and others in your group about reaching out to others with these questions: "How are you doing?" and "What's causing you stress?"

COMMITMENT

If you were a patient returning to my office for a follow-up appointment, I'd review what we learned about you and your health and remind both of us about the one or two simple things—one or two Biblical Prescriptions for Life—that you agreed to do as part of your journey.

There's no judgment involved here. If you missed doing them yesterday, then make sure not to miss doing them today. Don't get down on yourself. This journey is about direction—about moving consistently toward healing.

As you call your small group members today, remember to extend the same grace (kind favor and acceptance) to them. You and I often feel discouraged when we feel judged, whether by others or even by ourselves. Stop the negative self-talk and move forward. You can do this!

Refer to this chart on page 5. Keep track of your consistency. If you put in the effort, you will experience the results.

DAY 2

God's Original Design

Welcome to day two!

I'm so glad you've come back to the study. We have something very important to learn today that will provide one of the major keys to help us all benefit from Biblical Prescriptions for Life!

Yesterday we focused on stress, which manifests itself as a symptom such as pain. Something as lowly—pun intended—as your foot can land you in my cardiology office complaining of chest pain. I can't emphasize this concept enough: *When we use our bodies in ways that disregard their original design, we experience stress on our system and, sooner or later, a symptom develops.*

Remember: Living outside of our design > stress > stress chemistry > damage > symptom > and eventually, acquired disease. Is it really that simple? And if it is, can't we just begin to honor God's design in our life and everything will be perfect again? The answer is YES, although we (or at least as "perfect" as we can be in a sinful world). There is hope! We've been designed to be healthy and enjoy peace. The very best news is that there's someone waiting and eager to teach us how to get there.

Today, let's build on our understanding of design. How did the Creator design us to function?

It's evidence of our Creator that our feet are designed like they are. The arch is one of the strongest architectural structures known to man and you have one below each ankle! Think of the arches in the Roman aqueducts that still stand throughout Europe. Think of the arches that have kept many of the world's most famous ceilings in place for hundreds and even thousands of years.

Those wonderful arches imbedded in each foot distribute body weight and flex to absorb shock during movement. The five metatarsals and five tarsals in each foot articulate the movement so we can walk, run, jump, swim, climb and dance. Neural signals between thousands of pressure receptors communicate with your eyes and inner ear resulting in hundreds of physical micro adjustments per second—mini flexes of the small and large muscles in each foot—thus allowing us to balance while standing on solid rock or walking hundreds of feet above ground on a tight rope.

Try this—stand barefooted on a solid surface and pay attention to the almost imperceptible movements each of foot makes while the rest of your body remains motionless. Want another example? If you're able, balance on one foot and the movements of that foot will become very obvious! Amazing!

Like our feet, our entire bodies were created to live and perform at their fullest potential within a clear purpose and plan. I can almost hear you ask, "So, what is that purpose and plan, Dr. Marcum?"

Glad you asked. I'm going to stun you with the simplicity of the plan. And God is going to amaze you with magnificence of the plan. It's found in the first book of the Bible, Genesis, chapter 1. The Bible's verses are numbered so readers can navigate more easily within each of the 66 books.

> Then God said, "Let us make man in our image, after our likeness. And let them have dominion over the fish of the sea and over the birds of the heavens and over the livestock and over all the earth and over every creeping thing that creeps on the earth." So God created man in his own image, in the image of God he created him; male and female he created them.
>
> And God blessed them. And God said to them, "Be fruitful and multiply and fill the earth and subdue it, and have dominion over the fish of the sea and over the birds of the heavens and over every living thing that moves on the earth."
>
> And God said, "Behold, I have given you every plant yielding seed that is on the face of all the earth, and every tree with seed in its fruit. You shall have them for food. And to every beast of the earth and to every bird of the heavens and to everything that creeps on the earth, everything that has the breath of life, I have given every green plant for food." And it was so.
>
> And God saw everything that He had made, and behold, it was very good. And there was evening and there was morning, the sixth day. (Genesis 1:26-31)"

Now I want you to do something that will help you see the starting point of *Biblical Prescriptions for Life*. I want you to mark Genesis 1:26-31 with:

•   A triangle on each use of "God" and His pronouns
•   A circle around each reference to "man", "woman", mankind and their pronouns

Who made man and woman? _____

What was the design example used in the creation of man and woman?_____

What were the instructions given to man and woman? _____

Although we did not include it here, if you start reading the Creation account beginning in Genesis chapter 1 verses 1 through 31, you'll read about all six days of creation (God rested on the seventh day). Between the first and fifth days of Creation—days one through five—the Bible records for us that God "saw" (Hebrew = "ra'ah" to recognize or declare) that His work was "good" after each day had ended. On the sixth and final day of creation, God performs His crowning creative act by creating man and woman in His own image. Remember, He has created everything we know from *absolute nothing*. Here's how He considers the total of His Creation: "And God saw everything that he had made, and behold, it was very good. And there was evening and there was morning, the sixth day" (Genesis 1:31).

Did you notice the difference? He declared the total of His creative work, which culminated in the creation of mankind in His own image, to be *very* good. The world was "good." We—you and I—made the whole project "very good." I like that!

This was a time like no other on the Earth. Just the thought of this beautiful place designed from the ground up to serve a clear purpose (enjoying God and others in health and happiness) makes me feel at peace.

WRAPPING IT UP

If you try to look beyond the destruction man has brought upon himself and our planet, you can obtain a glimpse of how things used to be. Beautiful. Whole. Peaceful. Harmonious. Pure. This amazing creation—from the atoms that make fresh water to the galaxies circling throughout the universe—it was all very good! Then God gave us work to do. It amounted to farming and caretaking of the natural world. Our original job was to steward something given to us. And, even more glorious, He created us to be in a relationship with Him *and each other*. Without these relationships, there would be stress.

What an amazing journey you and I have begun.

LIVING IN COMMUNITY

How did you do connecting with someone from your small group yesterday? If you had a little trouble, here's some good news. Today is a brand new day! Why not make time to reach out and invest in a relationship with a fellow traveler on this journey toward healing. You can begin by asking that person what they thought of as they read about our original design and God's original plan for our lives.

BEING MISSIONAL

Do you know someone who may have an imbalanced view of God? Maybe they think He's an angry, judgmental old man. Maybe they think He is all-love and no power. Ask God to give you the opportunity today to talk with someone about the biblical concept that God created us for a relationship with Him.

COMMITMENT

I find patients experience the "aha" moment (that time when what you're learning suddenly makes sense in a special, lucid way) when they see the bigger picture.

Your cardiovascular system doesn't operate in a vacuum. It's connected to every other system of your body. As we'll learn in later chapters of Biblical Prescriptions for Life, it even goes farther than that. In fact, whole life healing and wellness goes well beyond us!

— DAY 3 —

Original Stress

I can't help it. It's overwhelming. I find encouragement and hope as I continue to study the incredible ways God designed us. Almost every day I'm discovering scientific evidence that demonstrates His healing ways *work* in the real world. I want to make His divine guidelines the treatments I share.

Are you ready to start putting two of the major *Biblical Prescriptions for Life* ideas together? Today we're going to begin to see how the painful symptoms that people like Michelle experience relate to God's original design. We'll start to see how symptoms indicate underlying unnatural, harmful conditions that can grow into life-threatening illness. And, we will move another day forward in applying God's solutions to our need for healing by following *His* Biblical Prescriptions for Life.

Let's review what we've learned together so far. These are the first steps.

- Modern medicine, treatments and technology play a valid role in acute care—they get us over the hump. There are great physicians, providers, and hospitals helping the healing process, especially in emergency situations.

- Presenting symptoms—i.e., chest pain, shortness of breath, elevated heart rate, high blood pressure—aren't the cause. They're the *result* of the cause.

- God made everything good. We were designed to live according to His plan. Inputs, physical or mental, contrary to that plan, puts stress on the system and sets in motion the potential for symptoms and disease.

Stop and think about that last point.

Something's wrong. You know it. I know it. Our bodies hurt. We get sick. We see people suffer with lifelong, chronic illnesses. We watch as people die. And it goes beyond our own skin and bones. We observe pollution in the environment, disharmony in relationships, and wars over ideology and resources. Most heartbreaking of all, we recognize wicked exploitation of the weak. This all leaves us asking, "Why? If God made everything very good, why is it painfully obvious that things are very, *very* bad? Why is our world so sick? Why are the rates of cancer, heart attacks, strokes, diabetes, obesity and mental health problems constantly on the rise?"

Read these two verses out loud to discover God's answer to that question:

"Therefore, just as sin came into the world through one man, and death through sin, and so death spread to all men because all sinned ... for sin indeed was in the world before the law [i.e., the Ten Commandments] was given" (Romans 5:12-13).

The original plan was to trust, obey, and love God. This plan was disrupted—the original stress. Then, disease set in.

Read the entire chapter of Genesis 3 reprinted here and mark:
- God and His pronouns with a triangle
- The serpent and his pronouns with a pitchfork (yes, that's a little campy and expected)
- Death with a large X
- Man, woman and their pronouns with "MK" for mankind
- Cursed with a rectangle

Now the serpent was craftier than any other beast of the field that the Lord God had made. He said to the woman, "Did God actually say, 'You shall not eat of any tree in the garden'?" And the woman said to the serpent, "We may eat of the fruit of the trees in the garden, but God said, 'You shall not eat of the fruit of the tree that is in the midst of the garden, neither shall you touch it, lest you die.'" But the serpent said to the woman, "You will not surely die. For God knows that when you eat of it your eyes will be opened, and you will be like God, knowing good and evil."

So when the woman saw that the tree was good for food, and that it was a delight to the eyes, and that the tree was to be desired to make one wise, she took of its fruit and ate, and she also gave some to her husband who was with her, and he ate. Then the eyes of both were opened, and they knew that they were naked. And they sewed fig leaves together and made themselves loincloths.

And they heard the sound of the Lord God walking in the garden in the cool of the day, and the man and his wife hid themselves from the presence of the Lord God among the trees of the garden. But the Lord God called to the man and said to him, "Where are you?" And he said, "I heard the sound of you in the garden, and I was afraid, because I was naked, and I hid myself." He said, "Who told you that you were naked? Have you eaten of the tree of which I commanded you not to eat?" The man said, "The woman whom you gave to be with me, she gave me fruit of the tree, and I ate." Then the Lord God said to the woman, "What is this that you have done?" The woman said, "The serpent deceived me, and I ate."

The Lord God said to the serpent, "Because you have done this, cursed are you above all livestock and above all beasts of the field; on your belly you shall go, and dust you shall eat all the days of your life. I will put enmity between you and the woman, and between your offspring and her offspring; he shall bruise your head, and you shall bruise his heel."

To the woman he said, "I will surely multiply your pain in childbearing; in pain you shall bring forth children. Your desire shall be for your husband, and he shall rule over you."

And to Adam he said, "Because you have listened to the voice of your wife and have eaten of the tree of which I commanded you, 'You shall not eat of it,' cursed is the ground because of you; in pain you shall eat of it all the days of your life; thorns and thistles it shall bring forth for you; and you shall eat the plants of the field. By the sweat of your face you shall eat bread, till you return to the ground, for out of it you were taken; for you are dust, and to dust you shall return."

The man called his wife's name Eve, because she was the mother of all living. And the Lord God made for Adam and for his wife garments of skins and clothed them. Then the Lord God said, "Behold, the man has become like one of us in knowing good and evil. Now, lest he reach out his hand and take also of the tree of life and eat, and live forever" therefore the Lord God sent him out from the garden of Eden to work the ground from which he was taken. He drove out the man, and at the east of the Garden of Eden he placed the cherubim and a flaming sword that turned every way to guard the way to the tree of life. (Genesis 3)

What did the Serpent want Eve to do? _____

Did the Serpent get God's instruction about the Tree of the Knowledge of Good and Evil right? _____

After God made Adam, He placed the man in the Garden of Eden to enjoy life and serve as a steward of all of God's creation. God put Adam in paradise. We can't even imagine it today with our limited understanding and blemished faculties.

Adam had everything to gain and untold wonders surrounding him not to mention the magnificence of living daily with the God of the universe! And this was just before God made the first woman Eve so Adam would know relationship on the most intimate terms. In light of God's cosmologically scaled generosity, God gave Adam a single request.

The LORD God took the man and put him in the Garden of Eden to work it and keep it. And the LORD God commanded the man, saying, 'You may surely eat of every tree of the garden, but of the tree of the knowledge of good and evil you shall not eat, for in the day that you eat of it you shall surely die.' (Genesis 2:15-17)

Did you catch *why* God gave this commandment? It was to prevent death! If Adam disobeyed the only restriction God gave him, Adam would die. He didn't need to understand why or even what death entailed. He was simply asked to trust and obey. This was part of the original plan.

How did God respond to the decisions and actions of Eve, the Serpent, and Adam? Make a list of the consequences.

Eve: _____

The Serpent: _____

Adam: _____

Did Adam and Eve die that day? Explain your answer. _____

Did Adam and Eve understand what death was? _____

Did they understand that the relationship with God and each other had been damaged? _____

Could they understand they were moving away from the original plan, damaging their bodies? _____

WRAPPING IT UP

God tells us in Romans 5.12-13 that through one man—Adam—sin (the original stress) entered the world and condemned all mankind. His sin condemned his children and grandchildren. In medical terms, we've all "inherited" the "sin gene" and with it, physical duress, illness, disease and death. This is a stressor causing real problems. We have inherited the consequences of living contrary to the original design. We've also inherited a dysfunctional relationship with God (we're born rebels who defy Him) and a potentially defective relationship with every other human being (we're genetically selfish and will use all means to get what we want and stay alive). This is what reptiles do. This is how their brain works. This endlessly selfish brain creates the stress chemistry.

How do you see this in the world around you? _____

How do you see it in yourself? _____

LIVING IN COMMUNITY

Your study group needs you. One way to live as we were created to live is by seeking and nurturing healing relationships. Your investment in the life of someone else brings you healing as it brings them healing. We'll learn more about that in sessions to come.

In the meantime, today is the day to make contact with at least one person on your list. If there's someone you haven't connected with yet, choose that person and get hold of him or her today.

BEING MISSIONAL

"So that's how stress began!" We've acclimated to a broken way of living and surviving in a diseased creation. Imagine the surprise on someone's face when you share that the stress we think is normal is not normal and there is a clear way to return to peace and healing.

COMMITMENT

How are you doing on your first Biblical Prescriptions for Life? Are you starting to recite the verses from memory? Can you get started with just a one or two word prompt? Are you finding that God is bringing these verses—these fundamental truths—to your mind when you find yourself in stressful situations?

Keep going. If you missed yesterday, make sure to practice today.

DAY 4

The Answer

Michelle felt as if her life was a total mess. She'd lost her job because she no longer fit the corporate image at the appearance-conscious legal firm she'd served faithfully for 20 years. She was ashamed of how she'd let herself go while rehabilitating her foot. She wasn't sleeping, was battling depression, and her foot wasn't healing properly! She'd gained enough weight to change her wardrobe several times over the course of a few years. She was on too many medications and was being treated by her general practitioner and five specialists. That's when she came to me with concerns about her heart.

Even though she felt like it, Michelle was not alone.

After reading the historical account recorded for us in Genesis chapter 3 yesterday, we've seen how stress entered the human race. We've seen how stress has entered all of creation. It has settled in our relationships. It stalks our livelihoods. And now millennia after the fall of mankind, the damage can be seen everywhere!

So where's the hope? Where is the prescription to fix the problem? Is the solution to all of these destructive symptoms really found in a pill or procedure?

I'm here to tell you the best news imaginable. It's even better than the news that God created us for a very good life: a life in perfect relationship with Him, experiencing whole-life health, relational harmony, and life-long healing. What's the *best* news? After our great-great-great (great, great…) grandfather Adam made a poor choice, God Himself provided the way back to paradise.

In infinite love, He provides:
- The path to healing and wholeness that we can start experiencing today.
- The final, ultimate healing that will last forever and will never again be forfeited.

How does He do that? Consider this amazing Bible passage: "So it is written: 'The first man Adam became a living being'; the last Adam, a life-giving spirit…the first man was of the dust of the earth, the second man from heaven" (1 Corinthians 15:45, 47). God Himself has brought redemption and healing into our world through Jesus Christ, the "second Adam." What a treatment for healing! What the first Adam failed to maintain, God's own perfect Son has remedied on our behalf. Jesus has undone the fall! And, in doing so, He has given His followers the free gift of eternal life: the ultimate and ever-lasting solution for all stress and resultant diseases.

Here we find the treatment for all ailments. Let's read how Romans 5.12-19 puts it. Mark:
- Adam with an A
- Jesus with a cross

Therefore, just as sin came into the world through one man, and death through sin, and so death spread to all men because all sinned—for sin indeed was in the world before the law was given, but sin is not counted where there is no law.

Yet death reigned from Adam to Moses, even over those whose sinning was not like the transgression of Adam, who was a type of the one who was to come.

But the free gift is not like the trespass. For if many died through one man's trespass, much more have the grace of God and the free gift by the grace of that one man Jesus Christ abounded for many. And the free gift is not like the result of that one man's sin. For the judgment following one trespass brought condemnation, but the free gift following many trespasses brought justification.

For if, because of one man's trespass, death reigned through that one man, much more will those who receive the abundance of grace and the free gift of righteousness reign in life through the one man Jesus Christ.

Therefore, as one trespass led to condemnation for all men, so one act of righteousness leads to justification and life for all men.

For as by the one man's disobedience the many were made sinners, so by the one man's obedience the many will be made righteous. (Romans 5:12-19).

Make a list of what we have in Adam compared to what we have in Christ.

In Adam	In Jesus

Take a good look at those lists.

There's no greater story of redemption! There can be no greater means of healing! We've been brought from death to life for eternity! And we can start experiencing this redemption right now as we follow Christ back to the Father's perfect design.

Read the next two passages out loud.

> For I consider that the sufferings of this present time are not worth comparing with the glory that is to be revealed to us. For the creation waits with eager longing for the revealing of the sons of God. For the creation was subjected to futility, not willingly, but because of him who subjected it, in hope that the creation itself will be set free from its bondage to corruption and obtain the freedom of the glory of the children of God.
>
> For we know that the whole creation has been groaning together in pains of childbirth until now. And not only the creation, but we ourselves, who have the firstfruits of the Spirit, groan inwardly as we wait eagerly for adoptions as sons, the redemption of our bodies. For in this hope we were saved. Now hope that is seen is not hope. For who hopes for what he sees? But if we hope for what we do not see, we wait for it with patience. (Romans 8:18-25)

Do you see the "pains of childbirth"? These pains are the symptoms we bear as we live under the stress of life. Can you relate to this?

Here comes the best news in health—the best news in the universe. Listen to how the story of the fall and its consequences ends for people in relationship with Jesus the returning King.

> Then I saw a new heaven and a new earth, for the first heaven and the first earth had passed away, and the sea was no more. And I saw the holy city, new Jerusalem, coming down out of heaven from God, prepared as a bride adorned for her husband.
>
> And I heard a loud voice from the throne saying, 'Behold, the dwelling place of God is with man. He will dwell with them, and they will be his people, and God himself will be with them as their God. He will wipe away every tear from their eyes, and death shall be no more, neither shall there be mourning, nor crying, nor pain anymore, for the former things have passed away.'
>
> And he who was seated on the throne said, "Behold, I am making all things new." Also he said, "Write this down, for these words are trustworthy and true."
>
> And he said to me, "It is done! I am the Alpha and Omega, the beginning and the end. To the thirsty I will give from the spring of the water of life without payment. The one who conquers will have this heritage, and I will be his God and he will be my son." (Revelation 21:1-7)

When we live in a way that is less than God's good and perfectly loving design, we live in a chemistry of stress. Do you have chest pain from a cascade of mounting stressors? Do you have debilitating, irreversible, life-threatening acquired disease? Do you have broken relationships? Jesus will make all things right in His time: our bodies, our minds, the plants, the animals, the environment, the joy in our work, and the wholeness in our relationships. Only *He* can perform this ultimate healing. He's the only one with the authority to heal.

WRAPPING IT UP

So this is the secret of true healing. It's not in modern medicine. It's not in therapeutic drugs. It's not in technology. It's not even within the skills and experience of today's well-intentioned healthcare professionals and researchers.

I want you to hear this very clearly. God sometimes uses all of these things. But please understand there is only one Ultimate Physician. Many times He heals in the here and now. He uses doctors and He uses modern medicine. Whether the medical team gives God the credit or not, all healing comes from Him alone. But *ultimate* healing—healing that springs from the very core of our being and addresses the cause of our diseases—comes from a right relationship with Him alone. When we are partaking in this relationship—this treatment—we're looking for Biblical recommendations to improve our entire life. We must be still and know the real source of healing.

LIVING IN COMMUNITY

Today, you and I have learned the single greatest truth in healthcare. It's the single greatest truth in any context. The key to health and wholeness is our relationship with the God who made us.

He made us for this relationship as well as relationships with one another. Make sure you call your study buddy today. Text everyone on the list. Connect with them. Do it! You will gain more than you can imagine in daily relationships with God and your fellow human beings, starting with the wonderful people on your journey through Biblical Prescriptions for Life.

BEING MISSIONAL

Do you know someone who is burdened—weighed down—with worry? Pray for them right now. Ask God for an opportunity and the right word or action that can enable you to place your shoulder under one corner of their burden and lift it with them in prayer.

COMMITMENT

There are only two days left in this first week of Biblical Prescriptions for Life. And although the first prescription included memorizing Bible verses, I hope by this point you're beginning to see the priority of getting our thoughts in line with God's design. Changes in belief precede changes in action. It's up to you to be honest with yourself in light of God's truth and commit to change. God is there to help give you the strength.

The good news is it's never too late. Start with your prescription right now and move forward on the journey towards healing.

DAY 5

Do You (Really) Want to be Made Well?

Imagine this: you schedule an appointment with my office. Maybe you want to make sure your cardiovascular system is functioning well. Maybe you have a symptom that is causing concern and you've finally carved some time out of your schedule to get it checked out. Whatever the reason, you've made the decision to get help.

In our first week together, I want you to think about your needs: the symptoms of your life. I also want you to realize where the true answers will come from: a relationship with God.

The theme is basically honesty and transparency. You won't start your journey to whole life health until you've faced reality. And you can't help your physician *help you* until you become brutally honest and transparent. This is a critical prerequisite to developing real relationships both with God and your fellow man. You can fake it, but you won't make it.

This week, we've been studying the Bible by looking for key words.

Today, we're going to use that study tool to look deeply and honestly at our beliefs and our subsequent behaviors. After all, every action you take is driven by a belief. If you don't hold your beliefs up to the perfect Word of God, your thinking will career from one error to the next and your lifestyle will start to reflect the absence of God's guidance.

The good news is that God wants to be in a relationship with us. This is the place—the only place—where our true needs are met. Are you ready for a relationship with Him? Are you ready for Him to do everything He wants to do in your life?

More than any other day this week, today's passage of God's word will probably dig into our motives, and that can be uncomfortable. By nature, we avoid discomfort. Our primitive brains motivate us to avoid painful stimuli, to seek pleasure, and to find nourishment. Today's discomfort, however, is good for us. So let's stop now and ask God to lead us into all truth, whether or not it hurts.

You might start like this, *"Father—thank you for wanting to speak to me today. I want to learn what You say about my health and my relationship with You. Thank You for Jesus making our relationship possible. And thank You, Holy Spirit for promising to lead me into all truth. Amen."*

Now—on to what the Ultimate Physician has for you and me today!

As you read this passage from the Gospel of John, chapter 5, please mark these words:
- "Jesus" and pronouns that refer to Him with a cross.
- "The sick man" and pronouns with a red circle.

After this, a Jewish festival took place, and Jesus went up to Jerusalem. By the Sheep Gate in Jerusalem there is a pool, called Bethesda in Hebrew, which has five colonnades. Within these lay a large number of the sick—blind, lame, and paralyzed — waiting for the moving of the water, because an angel would go down into the pool from time to time and stir up the water. Then the first one who got in after the water was stirred up recovered from whatever ailment he had. One man was there who had been sick for 38 years.

When Jesus saw him lying there and knew he had already been there a long time, He said to him, "Do you want to get well?"

"Sir," the sick man answered, "I don't have a man to put me into the pool when the water is stirred up, but while I'm coming, someone goes down ahead of me." (John 5:1-9)

- What was happening at the Pool of Bethesda in Jerusalem? _____
- Who was gathered and why were they there? _____
- What do we learn about the lame man? _____
- Why was this man hopeless? _____

In verse 6, the story reveals that Jesus saw the man and knew that he had already been there a long time. Amazing, isn't it? The Son of God chose the precise times in which He would perform His healings. He raised people from the dead on several occasions. Yet most of the people He healed had been suffering—suffering publicly—for a long time. You can read about His healing of the woman who'd endured 12 years of chronic bleeding (Luke 8:42-48) and the man who'd been blind from birth (John 9:1-7).

So, here at this public place of mysterious healing, a lame man has been waiting...and waiting, never anyone to help him. He was never able to get to the water in time before someone else received the healing. Day after day. Week after week. Month after month. Years had passed. He spent a lifetime watching others receive the freedom that for him was just out of reach.

That puts the question Jesus asks him in verse 6 in a very interesting context. Did the man still want to be healed or had he become accustomed to disappointment? Had he grown fatalistic in his prospects? Had he made friends with his infirmities? Had his illness become who he was? It was how he lived. There were undoubtedly friends and kind strangers who made sure he was clothed and fed without having to work to provide for himself. It made most of his life decisions pretty simple.

In light of all of this, *did he really want to be healed*?

We're not told why the lame man doesn't answer directly but we do hear his excuse. Jesus then simply, powerfully and effectively commands him, "Get up. Pick up your mat and walk!" No more excuses. No time for negotiation or doubt. Jesus, the Ultimate Healer, demonstrates His authority over everything by making a chronically lame man walk again. How? By commanding it to be so!

I've been completely transparent with you. Putting egos aside, the best any medical doctor can do is *practice* the healing arts for Jesus is the Ultimate Healer. Still, I think the question for you right now is the same simple yet profound question Jesus asked 2,000 years ago. "Do you want to be made well?"

Don't dismiss it too quickly. You're now beginning to understand your needs. Maybe this is one of your needs: a real, burning desire to actually be well. What are your needs? Jesus, in many instances starts the relationship by meeting a health need.

Truth is, I see patients every day who present with symptoms across the spectrum of severity. And this may shock you—but many of them don't really want to get better. How can I say this? Because I've witnessed their complete lack of effort to follow even the simplest, most critical instructions to save their lives. They either are not dealing honestly with their illness or they've already made up their minds that it's not worth the effort.

How about you? Do you want to be made well?

_____

_____

_____

WRAPPING IT UP

Yesterday we learned a secret of healing. The key is found in a relationship with God. In today's lesson, we found another secret: your willing participation is required.

Recite Mathew 11:28. What are you asked to do? Are you willing?

If you have not answered Jesus' question, this is the time to do it. Right now—before you move on with your day and get distracted by the many cares and concerns in your busy schedule—this is the right time to write your response. If you answer "yes"—are you ready to take the next step toward healing, even if it requires trust and effort? If you answer "no"—why? What is holding you back? Be specific and put it on paper in the space above.

Telling Jesus "yes" will put you on the path to healing no matter from where you're starting.

If you want to be made well, then you're ready to move forward, beginning next week with some very practical, simple, and scalable (tailored by you) steps. Yes, you can start immediately to experience a physical—and lifelong—change by incorporating Biblical Prescriptions for Life.

LIVING IN COMMUNITY

Remember, God made us for relationships—a real relationship with Him and real relationships with others.

Whatever you have decided today, you need to share it with your small group the next time you meet. If you are ready to go forward, you're going to need each other on the Journey. There will be need for encouragement and accountability. And there will be cause for celebration!

If you're not ready to go forward, don't judge (or be critical of) yourself. And don't walk away from real community. Everyone has doubts. Face them together in a grace-filled, accepting, non-judgmental time of discussion. But don't disconnect. Keep studying along with your group. In the coming days and weeks, you may find your desire to get on the path to healing overcomes any reluctance you're experiencing right now. The fact that you are reading this lesson suggests that you may have a hidden desire to be well. I hope so.

In fact—this is probably a really good time to share your thoughts with someone in your group.

BEING MISSIONAL

Make a list of people in your life who need God to work in their lives. Pray for them by name. Ask God to meet them right where they are in a way that would be unmistakably His.

COMMITMENT

The first week is coming to a close. We studied God's perfect plan for you and me as He intended life to be on this amazing planet. Then we studied how things went wrong. And we learned how things keep going wrong and getting worse every time we live in a way that's contrary to God's perfect design. This creates stress. All the while, the world is pulling us towards other options in healing.

Today, do your best to complete the Biblical Prescription for Life you chose to work on at the beginning of the week. Let God's promises and encouragement nourish your spirit and give you peace and strength.

DAY 6

The Third Secret

I deliberately titled today's study the *third* secret. If you've missed the first two secrets to embarking on the journey of whole-life health, I encourage you to stop here and review the preceding days. Yes, those two secrets are truly that important for they're foundational to everything else we'll learn and the Biblical Prescriptions for Life we're going to integrate into our lives. Remember: we started with the question, "How are you doing?" Understanding your needs and how to have them met is a key to Biblical Prescriptions for Life.

For review—

The First Secret to Healing: _____

The Second Secret to Healing: _____

The Third Secret to Healing is another Truth with a capital "T" you might not hear anywhere else in the healthcare world. It's a truth so counter to modern medicine that you might actually be shocked to hear it.

Remember, we were created to live in a perfect, healthy, intimate relationship with God the Father who created us. In His wisdom, His desire to bring us the most abundant joy and peace we'll ever know in this life is accomplished by following His perfect plan. And that plan includes a mostly overlooked element: rest.

Rest is so very instrumental to healing that it's at the very foundation of its own Biblical Prescription for Life. It's one of the greatest secrets to healing because God designed it to be. That's why I'd like to focus our time together today on making sure you get the most out of resting.

First—the "why."

God's Example to Us

Part of God's perfect plan for this creation includes following His example. In Genesis chapter 1, you remember that God Himself—the all-powerful, all-knowing, all-effective, never-tiring Creator of the universe created everything in a very specific order. And with the exception of the method He used to create man, He simply spoke everything into existence. Now that's power, power unlike anything you or I can imagine!

So this indescribably powerful Creator who made everything complete, very good, and exactly as He intended it to be does one more very remarkable thing on the seventh day of creation. We learn about it in Genesis chapter 2:1-3.

> Thus the heavens and the earth were finished, and all the host of them. And on the seventh day God finished His work that He had done, and He rested on the seventh day from all His work that He had done. So God blessed the seventh day and made it holy, because on it God rested from all His work that He had done in creation.

There it is. God *rested*.

Let that sink in for a moment. How many times is the word "rest" or its synonym used in just those three verses?

_____

Just from verses 1-3, what makes you think this fact is important to God? _____

Did He need to rest? _____ Was He tired? _____ Did someone tell Him to rest? _____ Did anyone or anything give Him the example of resting? _____ Of course the answers are "NO!" It seems God's rest is more than a physical rest. There's another reason for it.

God's Commandment to Us

Most of us westerners bristle at the thought of *anyone* commanding us to do *anything*. But remember, God created us. His commands aren't some arbitrary dictum. They are given for our benefit. We don't toss the owner's manual for our new car across the room and shout, "How dare they command that I change the oil every six thousand miles! How dare they tell me what grade of gasoline to use!" No. We eagerly study the manual and gladly follow the "commands" offered by the manufacturer because we want our car to last for miles and miles and miles.

The same holds true for the rules of good nutrition, good hygiene, and communicable disease prevention. There are principles—rules!—we need to follow in order to be healthy and whole. We can choose to disregard these principles, but we do so at our own peril. And the Person who gave us rest is alone worthy of our obedience. Remember, the One who commanded rest is the God who designed us and knows what is best for our system.

Let's look at Exodus 20, verses 8-11.

> Remember the Sabbath *(rest)* day, to keep it holy *(different; set apart)*. Six days you shall labor, and do all your work, but the seventh day is a Sabbath to the LORD your God. On it you shall not do any work, you, or your son, or your daughter, your male servant, or your female servant, or your livestock, or the sojourner who is within your gates.
>
> For in six days the LORD made the heaven and the earth, the sea, and all that is in them, and rested on the seventh day. Therefore the LORD blessed the Sabbath day and made it holy.

What Resting Says About God and About Us

The God of the universe designed us to rest and gave us His example to follow. Now, I can go into great depth about the physiological, emotional or intellectual benefits of resting—and we'll get to those in a later chapter—but suffice it to say the same Creator who designed and made us wants us to rest. Whether or not we understand all the details, *it still is a part of His perfect plan for us.*

When we follow that plan; when we rest, we're saying to God:

"I'm trusting your example, Lord" (Genesis 2:1-3).
"I'm following your instructions, Lord" (Exodus 20:8-11).
"I'm trusting that this is a means to restoration and healing, even if I don't understand, nor can explain the exact physiology, Lord" (Leviticus 25.4; fields must rest, we must rest).

"I'm agreeing that I'm not self-sufficient and must remind myself to trust You, Lord" (Hebrews 4.8-11).

Technology has now advanced to the point where we are beginning to scientifically prove the chemical and physiological benefits of rest. The treatment for the stress we have been talking about this week is rest. We need physical, mental, and spiritual rest. Rest is given to us and is a powerful treatment. When we come to God, He promises us the treatment of rest.

God has made rest important and tied it to our relationships with Him. Since it's important to Him, we need to make it important to us. That means we need to prepare a time, a place, and our hearts for rest.

Prepare a Time

If you have something you must to do—something you can't let slip or get pushed aside amidst the din of urgent matters, something you can forget or avoid—the best way to get it done is to make an appointment for it on your calendar.

The reason for this is simple: a to-do list changes with priorities. An appointment dedicates time. When something is important, there's no higher prioritization tool than making time for it. Time is the most precious thing we manage and we each have a very finite amount of it to manage. Serious about doing anything? Put it on your calendar. Serious about getting on the path to life-long whole life wellness? *Put rest on your schedule and keep the appointment.*

In the Bible you'll discover "the Sabbath"—the day of rest—from Genesis to Revelation. A Biblical Prescription for Life is to set aside a time for rest. *Plan for it today*—before you get too busy. While you're at it, put a time for rest on your calendar for the next seven weeks. That will get you all the way through this study. By then, you may have begun to realize what God wants all of us to know about rest. Again, make a date with the Ultimate Physician and don't be late to your appointment.

Prepare a Place

Resting means *not doing* the mundane, six-days a week routine. It *does mean* doing activities that recharge your energy in meaningful, relationship-building ways.

Please think wisely about things you can do that will interrupt your normal routine and give you rest while providing an investment in your relationship with God and others. This is between you and God. You'll have to decide if watching "The Game" qualifies as relationship building. Likewise, joining a small group of people in your neighborhood who are fixing a widow's roof as an act of self-sacrificial love may very well be one of the most restful ways to spend this special day.

Jesus told His critics that His acts of love and mercy were exactly the type of actions meant for the Sabbath. If you have any doubt, just ask Jesus to make it clear to you. Ask Him to give you peace as you choose ways to invest your day of rest. Remember, rest is healing and changes your physiology. If you broke your arm, you wouldn't keep throwing fastballs. So don't expect Sabbath rest to be the same ol' same ol'. The body and mind require rest that breaks routine of life and sets in motion the hidden powers of healing.

Prepare Your Heart

Preparing your heart is an important part of resting. Remember, rest is part of our relationship with God. It's a Biblical prescription to change our chemistry. Rest for that reason. Rest to know Him more. Trust Him even though you don't fully understand how "resting" works. Trust Him even though your list of things to do grows while you take this all-important break from the rush of life.

Rest to meet Him, to spend time with Him, to discern His perfectly loving instructions designed to make us healthier. Rest to invest in relationships that are meaningful and life affirming.

Then watch as God uses this Biblical Prescription for Life to change your physiology by taking away stress chemistry and bringing healing to your mind and body.

WRAPPING IT UP

God designed us to rest. He gave Himself as an example. Then He gave us rest as His gift and antidote for a diseased world. Again, the treatment for stress is rest. God has promised to give us rest. We must accept the treatment. We need the physical, mental, and spiritual rest.

This may be one of the most difficult Biblical Prescriptions for Life because it's so countercultural. To busy people living in a culture that is saturated with technology, overwhelmed with media, demands our 24/7 attention, and driven by the fear that feeds "the get-ahead-or-fall-behind" mania, rest might seem like the one prescription we could and even should justify skipping. But don't believe it! Don't believe the lies and rationalizations. Instead *rest*. Trust the One who made you.

Take a moment now to write down ways you can rest and break your routine. Make this a priority! _____

_____

LIVING IN COMMUNITY

I can't think of a better way to remind us of the need for community than learning about this purposeful day of rest. I've said it every day this week: God made us for relationships—a real relationship with Him and real relationships with others.

Right after you've scheduled your day of rest for the next seven weeks in your calendar, reach out to your study buddy and the people in your group. Maybe you can join them in their rest. Maybe they would like to join you in yours. Encourage each other. How can we rest? What does rest look like?

We're all on this journey together. God will see us through even when we start in different places and at different paces.

BEING MISSIONAL

Examine the list of people you've been building this week and invite one of them to join you for fellowship.

COMMITMENT

The first week is coming to a close. We studied God's perfect plan and how He intended life to be on this amazing planet. Then we studied how things went wrong and learned how things keep going wrong and getting worse every time we live in a way that's contrary to God's perfect design.

Today, it is especially fitting to complete the Biblical Prescription for Life you chose to work on at the beginning of the week.

Both memory verses are directly related to God's plan—and source—of rest for us all.

DAY 7

Your Day of Rest

Use this space to record notes about today's rest.

How did you invest it? _____

Where did you rest? _____

Did you join others in their rest? _____

Did you serve someone in an act of selfless love? _____

What did you learn about God today? _____

What did you learn about yourself today? _____

Did the people you have been praying for come to your mind and you prayed for them again?

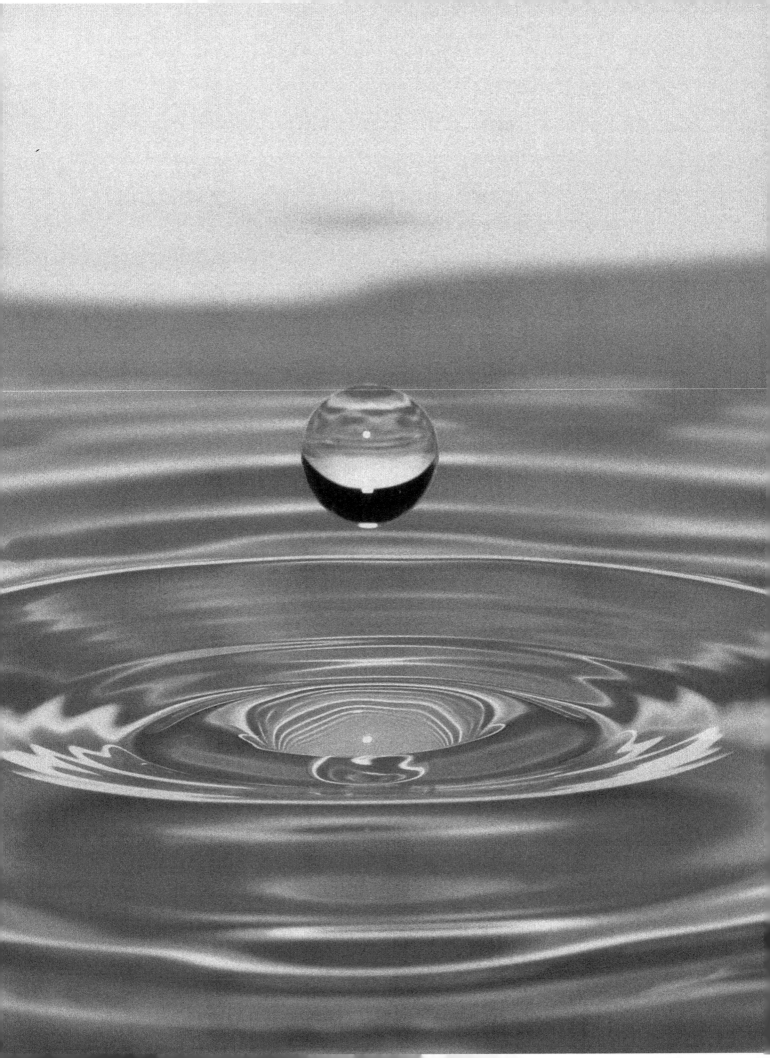

WEEK 2

Biblical Prescription for Life 1—Water for Your Body, Water for Your Soul

Feeling tired? Would you like to improve the function of every cell in your body? Consider this case history.

Mark was an excellent athlete and prided himself for staying healthy. He particularly enjoyed riding his bicycle long distances. One Sunday morning, in the heat and humidity of an August summer day, he set out on an eighty mile ride alone.

An hour into the journey, he realized he'd left his water bottles behind. He decided to venture on because he felt just fine. An hour later, he had a problem with the chain on his bike and had to stop. It took time for him to do the repairs. By now, it was starting to get hot and Mark was thirsty. Unfortunately, there were no houses or easy water access nearby so he decided to continue his ride.

By 11 a.m., the temperature was in the nineties and Mark's metabolism was increasing the core temperature of his body. Hyperthermia was setting in. He pressed on, but eventually had to stop because he'd become weak, was vomiting, and having trouble forming coherent thoughts.

Eventually, a car came by and the driver stopped to help the cyclist who now lay crumpled on the ground. The Good Samaritan wisely called for an ambulance and before long Mark was rushed to a hospital where a group of skilled doctors, nurses, and other care givers rushed to revive him. He was experiencing multi-organ failure from dehydration and hyperthermia.

When Mark arrived at the emergency room, his core body temperature was 105 degrees Fahrenheit. His blood pressure was 68/40, heart rate hovered around 160 beats a minute. His respiratory rate struggled at 30 breaths a minute. He was in a stupor and couldn't answer questions coherently. He was carrying no medical information and didn't even have a contact number on his person. A paramedic eventually found a drivers' license tucked away in one of the bags on his bike.

Mark was not doing well. He needed rapid improvement in every cell of his body.

Initial testing revealed that he was in renal failure with a condition called rhabdomyolysis that results from muscle breakdown. Fluids were quickly administered, cooling blankets applied, and support for every organ system was put into action. Because of renal failure, dialysis was initiated.

Mark didn't understand what was happening because he'd become delirious. His brain was simply not functioning.

Fortunately, after two weeks in the hospital, Mark recovered. Before he left, I reminded him that water is a fundamental necessity of life. Now he carries a fresh supply with him everywhere he goes.

This week, we're going to focus on how physical water is vitally important to our bodies. But there's an added benefit: when we're drinking enough water, our brains function more efficiently, thus helping us dip into the powerful stream of "Living Water" that God freely provides.

Many signs of dehydration match common physical symptoms of fear and panic. The stress chemistry is activated to keep the body alive. Dehydration to any degree is a stressor. When the two are combined, they strike the body doubly hard.

THE DOCTOR'S PRESCRIPTION

Here's how to calculate your pure, fresh, clean water intake need for each day:

- Weight in pounds divided by two equals needed ounces of water. (Example: If you weigh 150 pounds, you need to drink 75 ounces of water per day)

- Drink water until your urine becomes clear. Dark or clouded urine indicates dehydration.

Here are some beverages to reduce or remove from your daily intake:

Beverage	Calories per 12 oz/355 ml	Notable Chemical Compounds
Carbonated Soda/ Pop	400 average	Chemical acids in some sodas rob bones and teeth of calcium, weakening and discoloring them. High Fructose Corn Syrup (calorie-dense sweetener that's cheaper for manufacturers and more potent than sugar and possibly addictive) are empty calories which get stored as fat. Sodas contain many other chemicals we just don't need.
Caffeinated Coffee, Black	50 calories/cup	Caffeine, in excess, is a natural diuretic that draws precious water from your cells. It's also a vasodilator that increases blood flow, a stimulant that increases heart rate and perspiration, and a moderately addictive chemical toward which the body builds tolerance over time.
Coffee, with Cream & Sugar	500 calories/cup	All the dangers of caffeine with the added burden of dairy fat and sugar's empty calories.
Alcoholic beverages	calories that don't hydrate	Also addictive. Other organ systems may be affected.
Energy drinks	high in empty calories	Calories that do not hydrate as needed. Energy drinks may contain stimulants that increase metabolism artificially.

Biblical Prescriptions

Recite: John 4:13-14

Psalm 1:1-3

Jeremiah 17:7-8

(As the week goes on, hopefully you can commit these texts to memory.)

VIDEO GUIDE 2

What's Flowing Through You?

VIDEO (20 minutes)

Major Bible verses this week's Biblical Prescriptions for Life:

•   John 4:13-14; Psalm 1:1-3; Jeremiah 17:7-8

Who is Mark? What stands out to you about him? Is there anything in his life to which you can relate?

Level of activity _____

Dehydration symptoms _____

Lifestyle choices _____

We're learning about the chemistry of our amazing bodies and how we're designed to live in an environment based heavily on water—both inside and outside of us. What are the primary functions and benefits of water in our bodies?

Function	Benefit
_____	_____
_____	_____
_____	_____
_____	_____

Dehydration is serious—deadly serious. What are the risks at each range of dehydration?

Up to 5% _____

Up to 10% _____

Up to 15% _____

Over 15% _____

What can be our guideline for how much water we should drink each day?

_____

How many days a week is your fresh water intake less than those guidelines?

_____

Are there subtle ways that dehydration might be affecting your life?

_____

When we drink adequate amounts of water, less stress is put on the body: including the brain. Lack of water is a major stressor and activates stress chemistry. This stress chemistry is needed in an emergency like Mark was experiencing.

But, what if each one of us turns on this stress chemistry a little each day by not drinking enough water? Low level of dehydration will set in. Our body will compensate by activating a stress chemistry _cascade_. Epinephrine, cortisol, inflammatory mediators, and many more chemicals spring into action. The stress chemistry even changes our DNA. Because of the stress, our brain downshifts, sometimes making reasoning and problem solving a challenge.

Remember: we're trying to stay alive first. We are hardwired this way. Mark was glad his stress chemistry kept him alive until the cause of the stress was addressed. Our cognitive abilities will change to some degree under any stress. In Mark's situation, he could not even think.

Imagine walking in a desert, losing your source of water, and then beginning to see things that aren't there; you eventually would become incoherent, confused, and fearful. This is an extreme example. But this can happen in incremental degrees when we're dehydrated.

This may shock you: it's estimated that seven in ten people on this earth are dehydrated to some degree. Thankfully, the simple steps outlined here to improve our physical health will improve our mental health, decrease stress, and optimize our abilities to plug into our prefrontal cortexes ("upshift" our brains). This will allow us to grow more spiritually.

Group Discussion (20 Minutes)

- While viewing the video, what impacted you most? Why?

- Do you often reach for a favorite, non-water drink like a reward? Like a comforter? Like a pick-me-up?

- How can our drink choices reflect laziness or habit?

- How can our drink choices reveal an unhealthy appetite or even an addiction?

- How can our drink choices reveal a way we self-medicate? This may challenge our thinking, but have you ever reached for a drink that you thought would give you what only Jesus can give? What were you thirsty for?

And now with your group, finish this sentence—"_I want to change_____"

LIVING IN COMMUNITY

With the knowledge gained in Week One, we can start to experience the power of community in building relationships that are meaningful. In fact, each of us can take responsibility for reaching out to our study buddy and others in our group. It's not up to someone else. We all must make the effort.

Meaningful relationships—real relationships where we share each other's joys and pains, strengths and struggles—are a key need that God created within each of us. We can deny it. We may be afraid of being vulnerable but we all NEED relationships that are real, even if it's with one or two people.

As we continue through *Biblical Prescriptions for Life*, real, meaningful relationships are a key component to making changes that we can sustain for the duration of our journey to whole-life wellness.

The harmful effects of disconnected living can be seen every day in doctor's offices and hospital rooms. The long-term benefits far outweigh any short-term awkwardness or vulnerability you may experience.

Right now, ask your study buddy and other members of your small group how you can serve them this week as you and they integrate this powerful Biblical Prescription for Life.

Name	The Best Way I Can Care for Them	Mobile Number

INDIVIDUAL REFLECTION

Answer this question: As I listened to my friends and companions, what was my top-level take-away message from this weeks' time together? Write your response here: _____

BEING MISSIONAL

Water. Cold, clean water. Knowing what you know, imagine the physical and spiritual significance of going out of your way to bring a glass or bottle of water to someone this week. When Jesus returns and commends His believers, He will say. "...as you did it (*gave a drink to someone who was thirsty*) to one of the least of these my brothers, you did it to me" Matthew 25.40.

Just think, in a service as simple as giving someone a glass of water, we can change chemistry. We become loving, not selfish. Being selfish is a stay-alive, lower brain stress act, which moves our brains and health in the wrong direction.

COMMITMENT

Biblical Prescriptions for Life are simple, sustainable, and scalable changes you can make today that will bring real improvement to your life. Living life according to our Creator's plan will infuse wellness into your body from the inside out. Following God in faith, and performing these simple changes, will give you the healing tools needed to perhaps change your body to the point where your doctor can eliminate a prescription medication!

Remember, a prescription medication only treats one or two chemical pathways. Changing your life and brain by drinking water affects the entire system and often addresses the cause of a problem.

Last week, you started making simple changes. You documented them on a page. If you haven't already done so, transfer those notes to a page where you can keep a running, personal, Biblical Prescriptions for Life—a record that you plan to keep throughout the entire course. By the completion of your time together—with God's power and the support of your community—you'll discover that you've changed your life in simple, sustainable, and powerful ways.

For this our second week, here are Biblical Prescriptions for Life to add to your discipline from week one. Then tell yourself: "This week, I am going to ADD and FOLLOW at least one of the simple Biblical Prescriptions for Life." Place a checkmark on each day that you accomplish your goal:

I commit to	Biblical Prescription for Life	Day 1	2	3	4	5	6	7
	Read aloud 5x each day. Practice, memorize & recite							
	John 4:13-14 *"Jesus said to her, 'Everyone who drinks of this water will be thirsty again, but whoever drinks of the water that I will give him will never be thirsty again. The water that I will give him will become in him a spring of water, welling up to eternal life.'"*							
	Jeremiah 17:7-8 *"Blessed is the man who trusts in the Lord, whose trust is in the Lord. He is like a tree planted by water, that sends out its roots by the stream, and does not fear when heat comes, for its leaves remain green, and is not anxious in the year of drought, for it does not cease to bear fruit."*							
	Psalm 1:1-3 *"Blessed is the man who walks not in the counsel of the wicked, nor stands in the way of sinners, nor sits in the seat of scoffers, but his delight is in the law of the Lord, and on His law he meditates day and night. He is like a tree planted by streams of water that yields its fruit in its season, and its leaf does not wither. In all that he does, he prospers."*							
	Keep a drink journal for each day of the week.							
	Drink _____ ounces of fresh, clean water each day.							
	Remove one serving of _____ each day of the week							

If you missed a session or want to review one, go to biblicalprescriptionsforlife.com to stream this week's audio and video.

DAY 1

There's No Way to Hide Dehydration

Sandy came to the office a few weeks ago with a new symptom. She was having "funny poundings" in her chest—something she'd never experienced before. These sensations were, understandably, scaring her. Thankfully, she wasn't passing out. Previously, she'd gone to the emergency room, where she received blood tests, an EKG, and a chest x-ray. All were normal! She was 38 years old with two teenagers living at home.

When she came to see me, I placed a monitor on her and ordered an echocardiogram of her heart. While her heart strength was normal, the test did show numerous PVC's (abnormal beats from the bottom part of the heart). She seemed a little better when I explained that what she was experiencing was not dangerous. Then we started talking about how any stress—no matter how small—could increase the production of epinephrine that could, in turn, generate the PVC's. She admitted taking in energy drinks, but said she slept well and wasn't in pain. All of her labs and electrolytes were normal. She was not taking medications, diet pills, or caffeine that could raise the stress chemistry. She had a healthy relationship with her husband and was getting adequate rest. What was going on?

Then, I asked her about her water intake. Guess what? She wasn't drinking water.

Long story short, she increased the amount of water she drank each day and completely eliminated sodas from her diet. When she came back for a follow-up visit, she wore a big smile on her face and I knew immediately she was feeling better! "I never understood how important water was till I discovered how well I felt once I made it a priority," she told me. With this change of liquid intake, her PVC's quickly vanished.

Finding the *cause* of a symptom is much more rewarding than just treating a symptom. A common medical treatment in Sandy's case would've been to prescribe a beta-blocker and then monitor her regularly for side effects of the medication. Who wants that?

When a patient returns for a follow-up visit, I can discern within moments whether or not they've been sticking to the plan.

- What is their countenance like?

- Will they make eye contact with me?

- Do they remember what we talked about?

- Can I see a change in their appearance, in their posture, or in the way they walk or move?

- Are they enthusiastic about results?

- Are their vitals (weight, blood pressure, heart rate) different?

Sometimes as we talk, I discern why they've not stuck with my plan.

- Maybe they'll say, "I'm trying to overcome a crisis in their life,."

- Are they really committed to moving forward on their journey to health? Amazingly, some aren't!

- Are they committed to working with God on achieving a real and lasting change?

- Are they trying to do too much too quickly?

- Are they specific about challenges they've faced as they've put a Biblical Prescription for Life into practice?

- What are they learning about themselves in the process?

Knowing this, if you were wearing a white exam jacket, what would you perceive when *you, the patient*, walked into the office?

How would you encourage *you the patient* to stick to the plan and trust God as you change one step at a time?

I've found that most people respond positively to encouragement blended with clear, simple actions. The way your body responds will be evidence that the Biblical Prescription is working. The relationship you're cultivating with God will give you the power and encouragement to make any necessary changes.

We're getting to the basic steps that lead to health. Even though these steps may sound simple, seven out of ten people in this world are not drinking enough water and, as a result, are not enjoying the benefits.

This week we're going to do some very simple, very profound things in addition to drinking water. We're going to:

- Focus on trusting the Ultimate Physician.

- Focus on what God has to say about water.

- Journal our daily drink habits.

- Start drinking more pure, fresh, clean water.

- Reduce or, completely remove our consumption of less-than-healthy drinks.

Are you ready for change? Are you ready to take the next step on your journey toward healing and whole-life wellness?

Please keep this in mind: lack of water is a stressor activating the negative stress chemistry that generates endless health problems. If you keep this in your thoughts, hydrating with water will soon become second nature.

Now let's do the next Biblical Prescription for Life together.

Read the following two verses found in the book of Psalms, chapter 1, verses 1-3. Read this passage out loud so you can hear the words.

> Blessed is the man who walks not in the counsel of the wicked, nor stands in the way of sinners, nor sits in the seat of scoffers; but his delight is in the law of the Lord, and on his law he meditates day and night. He is like a tree planted by streams of water that yields its fruit in its season, and its leaf does not wither. In all that he does, he prospers.

This is an important and powerful metaphor; so important that God uses it to set the tone of the entire book of Psalms. It's so important and descriptive to a life of trusting God, that He repeats Himself in the book penned by Jeremiah.

In Jeremiah, chapter 17, verses 7-8 we read,

> Blessed is the man who trusts in the Lord, whose trust is the Lord. He is like a tree planted by water, that sends out its roots by the stream, and does not fear when heat comes, for its leaves remain green, and is not anxious in the year of drought, for it does not cease to bear fruit.

Both passages describe the same person.

- What are the beliefs and actions of this "blessed" person?

- To what is the person God who trusts God likened?

If you've traveled to the Middle East (or the U.S. southwest), you understand that water is the one thing that's more precious than oil. No one can take it for granted. No one can live without it. Those truths apply to all of us no matter where we live, but it is geographically apparent in the deserts of the world.

After reviewing the texts above, answer these questions:

Does God promise that droughts won't come? _____

What does He promise? _____

How do we hydrate our bodies in these types of life situations? _____

What's the meaning of this metaphor? _____

Is there something we need to do to benefit from this promise? _____

Our Ultimate Physician is speaking to us. Do you have something to say to Him? It might be that you are having a difficult time trusting Him. It might be that there are beliefs and habits that you're holding onto that go so deep you're not sure you can stop them. This would be a great time to talk to Him honestly and directly. He wants to communicate with us so He can help us even more.

WRAPPING IT UP

Last week we learned about what I call the "Three Secrets of Healing." 1. God created us for authentic relationship with Himself. 2. We must be willing participants in our healing and wellness. 3. God created rest for our benefit—something we disregard at our own peril.

Today, we learned about our necessity for water. God teaches us about water and trusting Him with an inseparable context. To be "watered"—or hydrated and experience all the benefits that entails—we must trust Him regardless of what anyone else may say. Water keeps us growing and functioning on a cellular level. We need physical and spiritual water for optimal physical functioning. This is how we were designed.

Trusting God at His word and following His words are a fundamental Biblical Prescription for Life, just as fundamental as...water. There's also evidence-based science that reveals that measurable physical changes take place in us as we worship. I will detail this in Week Six.

LIVING IN COMMUNITY

Hopefully, you've begun to experience community in your study. If so, keep the momentum going by contacting your study buddy with an encouragement *today*. Remember, God made us for relationships—a real relationship with Him and real relationships with others. You and I are half of any human relationship.

BEING MISSIONAL

Is there someone you know who could use a literal drink of water? Perhaps bringing a cold bottle of water to a co-worker today will be the start of a healthy relationship. Maybe offering one to your child as he or she works or plays would demonstrate your love. Either way, it's a valuable, healthful conversation starter and a true act of love.

COMMITMENT

You've embarked on a journey. I want to emphasize that your path will have milestones and that, along the way, we'll identify some harmful things to drop and healthful things to adopt. We'll commit, to ourselves and our community, to keep these changes for the rest of our lives. And when we fail (not "if"), we'll encourage ourselves, our study buddy and others in our small group—to dust ourselves off, ask God for a fresh supply of His powerful help, and move on.

Today, continue doing the 1-3 Biblical Prescriptions for Life you adopted last week and start working on the 1-3 the Biblical Prescriptions for Life you chose to address this week. The simplicity of each Biblical Prescription for Life makes it easy to add and then sustain them. Keeping them as you move forward creates real, lasting wellness in your lives.

I commit to	Biblical Prescription for Life	Day 1	2	3	4	5	6	7
	Read aloud 5x each day. Practice, memorize & recite:							
	John 4:13-14 *"Everyone who drinks of this water will be thirsty again, but whoever drinks of the water that I will give him will never be thirsty again. The water that I will give him will become in him a spring of water welling up to eternal life."*							
	Jeremiah 17:7-8 *"Blessed is the man who trusts the Lord, whose trust is the Lord. He is like a tree planted by water, that sends out its roots by the stream, and does not when heat come, for its leaves remain green, and is not anxious in the year of drought, for it does not cease to bear fruit."*							
	Psalm 1:1-3 *"Blessed is the man who walks not in the counsel of the wicked, nor stands in the way of sinners, nor sits in the seat of scoffers, but his delight is in the law of the Lord, and on His law he meditates day and night. He is like a tree planted by streams of water that yields its fruit in its season, and its leaf does not wither. In all that he does, he prospers."*							
	Keep a drink journal for each day of the week.							
	Drink _____ ounces of water each day.							
	Remove one serving of_____ each day of the week.							

I commit to	Biblical Prescription for Life	Day 1	2	3	4	5	6	7
	JOURNAL							
	Number of servings of soda							
	Number of servings of black coffee							
	Number of servings of coffee with cream and/or sugar							
	Number of servings of milk (____% fat)							
	Number of alcoholic drinks consumed							
	Number of servings of pure, fresh, clean water							

Drinks to limit:

- Carbonated beverages – most popular soft drinks, etc.

- Excessive coffee and additives, alcohol, sugary drinks, and energy drinks with sugar.

DAY 2

Water Cleanses Us Inside and Out

It doesn't matter where I am. I can be at the pool during a swim meet for my kids. I can be at the grocery store. I can be at church. I can even be in my office. No matter where I am, once people discover I'm a doctor, I get this question more often than I can count: "Dr. Marcum, what's the one thing I can do to improve my health *today*?"

Sometimes I answer this question *with* a question. "Do you smoke?" "Do you drink alcohol?" If they answer yes to either or both of those, then I recommend they stop those dangerous behaviors immediately, no questions asked.

If they answer no to both, then I tell them the one thing they can do to improve heart health immediately is to make sure that they're drinking enough pure, fresh water each and every day. Water has been a building block of any successful society. Cities were built around water. Commerce depended on water. In some places, just getting drinking water was a major task. That particular problem still exists in many parts of the world. Yet, as time has passed, water has become deemphasized, except for use in daily showers.

Why is water so valuable?

1. **Water is necessary in cellular metabolism.** Inside the cell, water is used within the cell's organelles (functional structures like mitochondria and vacuoles) in the process of converting glucose to energy. At the end of metabolism, outgoing water carries metabolic waste back into the blood stream where it is eliminated. Basically water is essential for the cell to function normally.

2. **Water is necessary to clean the surface of the body from dirt and contaminants.** Even with today's high tech chemical cleaners and antibacterial compounds, water is still the number one ingredient by volume.

3. **Water is needed by plants, which give us oxygen and is an energy source**. No water. No plants. No nutrients for our bodies.

Whether a person is well hydrated is one of the first assessments I make about a patient. Yet, even more important to whole-life healing and wellness is spiritual water. God is once again using the natural world to demonstrate a spiritual truth. Do they have Living Water as well? Here are three very good reasons for this question:

1. **Spiritual water is necessary for our spiritual metabolism.** It carries needed stress reducers, encouragement, love, and purpose directly to where it's needed most. Worship changes the chemical and physical aspects of our brains and shifts us from being like the animals to knowing our Creator God. This gives us the ability to move from selfishness to love.

2. **We need spiritual cleansing to become a child of God.** Our great forefather Adam acted unwisely. His rebellion caused a change in our very DNA that hardwired death and disease into our race and separated us from God. To be cleaned of this "dirt," we need cleansing water. This cleansing is called *salvation*.

3. God provides a way for us to be cleansed every time we act selfishly. Selfishness changes our chemistry because it's contrary to the original plan. Stress chemistry is activated. But our daily cleansing with God's Holy Spirit removes the sin and brings about maturity in Christ. This process is called *sanctification*.

We understand that our actions may hurt our relationship with God. When this relationship is damaged, our physical body is damaged as well. Remember we were made to be in harmony with our creator. Living outside this design is a stressor.

4. Living Water is essential to our growth and eternal well-being. Without God's Spirit flowing through us, we have no power for our eternal growth.

Spend a moment and let the parallels of physical water and spiritual water sink in. Is God speaking to you about both physical and spiritual water? Write down how you feel.

_____

Being washed physically clean is a powerful, memorable metaphor for having our spiritual "dirt" removed. We are all people in need of cleaning. God is the loving Father who rescues us from our contaminated, dirty condition. He then provides nourishment and power for our physical and spiritual life.

In each of the following passages, mark the following:

- "water" and its synonyms (use a blue oval)

- "clean" (the adjective) and "to be cleaned" (the verb phrase) including "removal of dirt," "wash" and their synonyms (use a blue rectangle). Note that "baptize" and "sprinkle" literally mean, "to wash."

"I will sprinkle clean water on you, and you shall be clean from all your uncleanness, and from all your idols I will cleanse you" (Ezekiel 36:25).

"Therefore, brothers, since we have confidence to enter the holy places by the blood of Jesus, by the new and living way that he opened for us through the curtain, that is, through his flesh, and since we have a great priest over the house of God, let us draw near with a true heart in full assurance of faith, with our hearts sprinkled clean from an evil conscience and our bodies washed with pure water. Let us hold fast the confession of our hope without wavering, for he who promised is faithful. And let us consider how to stir up one another to love and good works, not neglecting to meet together, as is the habit of some, but encouraging one another, and all the more as you see the Day drawing near." (Hebrews 10:19-25)

"Baptism, which corresponds to this, now saves you, not as a removal of dirt from the body but as an appeal to God for a good conscience, through the resurrection of Jesus Christ." (1 Peter 3:21)

"We were buried therefore with him by baptism into death, in order that, just as Christ was raised from the dead by the glory of the Father, we too might walk in newness of life." (Romans 6:4).

"And now why do you wait? Rise and be baptized and wash away your sins, calling on his name." (Acts 22:16)

"And Peter said to them, 'Repent and be baptized every one of you in the name of Jesus Christ for the forgiveness of your sins, and you will receive the gift of the Holy Spirit.'" (Acts 2:38)

Baptism (sprinkling with or immersion in water) symbolizes our eternal decision to follow Jesus and trust him for the forgiveness of our sins that separate us from God.

What is the connection between water, washing, and baptizing and our condition before God?

_____

Now, complete this chart listing what God's Word teaches about water and being cleansed.

What water & cleaning gives or removes...	...so that we have this new characteristic or benefit
_____	_____
_____	_____
_____	_____
_____	_____
_____	_____

Now, go back to each passage and single-underline the person who is doing the cleansing and double-underline the person being cleansed.

Who does the giving or cleansing? _____

Who receives the gift or gets cleansed? _____

What is God saying to you as you consider what you have learned so far today? Pause to reflect here and record your thoughts before you move on. _____

WRAPPING IT UP

This idea of needing God to cleanse us—to forgive us from wrongs—is both an eternally and immediately important health issue. This happens in the brain. We need this cleansing to remove the toxins and dirt from our life. This will help our stress chemistry. This will lead us away from damaging selfishness and toward healing love.

If you've never asked God to forgive and cleanse you from your sin, this may be the largest and most important issue at hand. Jesus is the Living Water. If you agree that you need Living Water and want to trust Him for this most important ingredient in your life, stop right now and tell Him that you want to accept His gift.

When God brought me to this simple realization, I was only ten years old. I spoke to Him in a very childlike prayer straight from my heart. And praise God, He heard me! If this is your desire, you might offer a prayer something like this:

"Father God, I know that I have disobeyed Your good, perfect, and loving instructions for my life. I know I have lived for myself instead of for You. Please forgive me. Please adopt me as Your eternal child. Please let me know You as my perfect Father and Jesus as my Savior and King. I want to live for You. I want to obey You. Please lead me into Your perfect plan."

If you have prayed this to God just now—I'm *thrilled* for you! You are officially on the path to eternal life. Welcome to the family! Just think. You are now drinking both physical water *and spiritual* water.

LIVING IN COMMUNITY

Today would be a great day to talk about cleansing with your *Biblical Prescriptions for Life* small group leader. Plan a time to text or call them today. Don't miss this opportunity to share what God is teaching you. Also don't forget to drink water—the physical kind. This will help you reduce stress and improve the function of every cell in your body. This will also help you communicate better with your source of Spiritual Water.

BEING MISSIONAL

The truth is that each of us needs to be cleansed from our physical and spiritual dirt. This is an eternally significant issue. Some people will understand. Some won't. Others will celebrate this freedom with you. Still others may ridicule the idea or oppose it vehemently. Ask God to direct you to the right people to share today's lesson. Point out the importance of drinking physical water first and, if the door opens, talk about Spiritual Water. Be thankful for the gift of water. If this is your starting place on the new, cleansed life in Jesus, I encourage you to share it with your small group leader first for his or her loving, prayerful guidance.

COMMITMENT

Are you beginning to see how your thoughts and beliefs are changing as you put Biblical Prescriptions for Life into practice? Memorization of God's word and simple changes in drinking choices are healthy habits. This is a journey and we're all on it together! Your spiritual and physical well being are inextricably connected.

Keep moving forward. If you didn't complete your Biblical Prescriptions for Life commitment yesterday, don't worry. Instead, accept the grace that God offers. Dust yourself off and practice them today!

• Journal your drink choices in your daily chart.

• Remind yourself of your other simple action steps and complete each one that you've committed to practice today.

- Pay close attention to how your body responds. Have your biometrics changed yet? *"Water* does a body good!"

- Your physical and Living Water will result in chemical changes.

- Make a neural connection. When you drink water, also remember the body's thirst for Spiritual Water.

DAY 3

Cleansing is Humbling in the Most Beneficial Way

Have you noticed that you like to do things *your* way?

Joann came to the office and said she was feeling just terrible. I'd known Joann for years and she wasn't a complainer. She's a young eighty-six and a little forgetful sometimes.

During our visit, she described a dizzy feeling every time she changed positions. She also complained of no energy and a racing heart. Her skin was dry and her blood pressure was 80/60. This was low for her. Her daughter-in-law asked her to come in for evaluation after a bout with diarrhea the week before, but Joann refused. She wanted to do things her way.

During that bout, she hadn't been drinking much water. One of the medications she was taking was a diuretic that is used for lowering blood pressure but also removes fluid from the body.

Well, to make a long story short, this medication had pulled water and potassium from her body. Now she was severely dehydrated with dangerously low potassium levels. Every cell in her body was affected. Her stress chemistry was doing the best job it could by increasing her heart rate to keep the blood pressure up. But she needed help and she needed it *now*!

Joann agreed to be admitted to the hospital for intravenous hydration and promised not to take the fluid pill if she were ill and not drinking water.

Do you believe you are the capable boss of your life, the best captain of your destiny? It's seemingly hardwired into us, to be independent, self-reliant, individualist, and full of pride.

Don't get me wrong. Self-respect is healthy. When we don't accept a lifestyle of poor choices and failure and, instead, work to improve ourselves and our service to others—that's not only productive, it's also showing genuine self-respect. When we don't let people abuse us, when we don't give into our base desires of laziness, greed or gluttony, when we don't settle for substandard because we value the preciousness God has placed on each of us as a person—that's agreeing with how God views us. And it's healthy.

Sometimes, we don't want to inconvenience others. Oftentimes, it's because we want to be self-reliant, to do things our way, to not humble ourselves by expressing our need to another person. This is self-sufficiency. But, when we place those attributes before the loving commands of our Holy God that becomes self-righteousness and is anything *but* healthy.

That brand of self-righteousness can be extremely detrimental. When we think we've arrived, we're most at risk to fall. When we think we're better than our fellow man, we lose touch with our humanity. When we think we're good enough on our own merit, we're deceiving ourselves. When we hold an inflated view of ourselves and judge everyone else by our own standard, we make ourselves to be god.

When we're thinking self-righteously, we're tempted to look down on people who are failing. We may even harbor judgmental thoughts against people who ask for help or depend on others more than we think we need to. "What's wrong with them?" we scoff. "They must deserve this." "Ugh, I'm so glad I'm not like that person!"

Because the contaminated DNA, which we inherited from Adam, leads to a self-centered predisposition, we often won't humble ourselves to the point of acknowledging our need for God to cleanse us from our inherited guilt. Think about how difficult it can be to say you're sorry to a friend or loved one. Think about how rare it is to see someone ask someone's *forgiveness* for a wrong committed against them. When was the last time you said, "I'm sorry"?

In fact, if we were totally honest, we would prefer to be worthy and acceptable on our own instead of needing Jesus to cleanse us. Yes, this desire to be in right standing with God on our own merit—is what the Bible calls "self-righteousness." It's an attempt to say, "I don't need Living Water. I can do things my way and come out just fine. I don't need a healer!"

You and I aren't the first to wrestle with this humbling need to be cleansed. Jesus' disciples expressed self-righteousness after living with and learning from Him for three years! During the Last Supper—Jesus' final meal with His disciples—they all gathered in the Upper Room before the Jewish Passover Festival. It was there that Jesus' confronted their self-righteousness directly. He knew this was a fatal disease needing immediate treatment. They may not have been aware of their condition because the disease of pride is a master at covering its tracks.

Listen to the story as recorded in John 13:1-11:

> It was now the day before the Passover Festival. Jesus knew that the hour had come for him to leave this world and go to the Father. He had always loved those in the world who were his own, and he loved them to the very end. Jesus and his disciples were at supper. The Devil had already put into the heart of Judas, the son of Simon Iscariot, the thought of betraying Jesus. Jesus knew that the Father had given him complete power; he knew that he had come from God and was going to God. So he rose from the table, took off his outer garment and tied a towel round his waist. Then he poured some water into a basin and began to wash the disciples' feet and dry them with the towel round his waist. He came to Simon Peter, who said to him, "Are you going to wash my feet, Lord?"

Jesus answered him, "You do not understand now what I am doing, but you will understand later."

Peter declared, "Never at any time will you wash my feet!"

"If I do not wash your feet," Jesus answered, "you will no longer be my disciple."

Simon Peter answered, "Lord, do not wash only my feet, then! Wash my hands and head, too!"

Jesus said, "Those who have had a bath are completely clean and do not have to wash themselves, except for their feet. All of you are clean—all except one." (Jesus already knew who was going to betray him; that is why he said, "All of you, except one, are clean.")

What was Jesus saying to them and us about cleansing?

Jesus used the natural world—washing of dirty feet—to explain the spiritual world. Cleansing water is important to wash away the dirt of pride and selfishness. Physical water is important to maintain the body.

One of those disciples in the Upper Room during the Last Supper was John. John wrote the Gospel of John and several other New Testament books. In the book called First John, chapter 1 verses five through seven, he writes:

This is the message we have heard from him and proclaim to you, that God is light, and in him is no darkness at all. If we say we have fellowship with him while we walk in darkness, we lie and do not practice the truth. But if we walk in the light, as he is in the light, we have fellowship with one another, and the blood of Jesus his Son cleanses us from all sin.

From this passage, we learn that Jesus is the Living Water and *that* water changes us. These are real structural and chemical changes in our body. Cleaning changes us! We move from putting our interests first (selfishness), to putting the interests of others above our own (love). We confess our shortcomings, acknowledge our disease, and ask the Great Physician for treatment. He offers His prescription of Living Water and when we accept that treatment, healing begins.

What can you do right now to improve your relationship with God? If you don't know, just bow your head and ask Him. He's listening. And, when you drink your next glass of physical water, remember to ask for a loving dose of Living Water as well.

WRAPPING IT UP

We covered eternal, life-transforming truths from the Bible yesterday and today:

1. **We are born with bad DNA and need a treatment for that dangerous condition**. We know where the treatment is found. This is a whole-person washing—figuratively inside and out. God who alone can cleanse us makes our whole person—body, soul, mind and spirit clean.

2. **After God cleanses us and gives us salvation, we still might disobey Him and give in to our selfish desires.**

    These acts re-separate us from Him. That's why we must allow Him to "wash our feet" each and every day.

Agreeing with God that we need Him to clean us is an act of humility. But without this humility, Jesus tells us in Matthew chapter five that we'll never enter Heaven,

| "Blessed are the poor in spirit, for theirs is the kingdom of heaven" (John 5:3).

This means literally: "Oh the blessed, joyful condition of the person who recognizes that they need Living Water to save them."

Let that thought sink in for a moment. Then ask God to help you trust Him as you consider this truth.

LIVING IN COMMUNITY

There's more at stake here than your physical health. When you have a moment, call your small group leader and celebrate that realization with him or her. Ask questions. Ask about how they came to trust God. Ask them how God is changing their life today since they first went to Jesus with that simple act of humility.

BEING MISSIONAL

Is there someone you know who will not believe what God says about their need to be cleansed? Pray for that person right now. This realization and acceptance is a supernatural breakthrough that we may witness. We sometimes get to encourage them with our personal experience finding God's unconditional, non-judgmental love at the end our confession and repentance. As you pray together, remember the power our God has to change the lives of others.

COMMITMENT

- Are you trying your best?

- When you give in to an old habit, do you dust yourself off and try again?

- If so—are you making progress? Do your best today and be thankful that you're breathing, thinking and drinking life-giving water along the journey to healing and whole-life wellness.

- Journal your drink choices in your daily chart.

- Remind yourself of your other simple action steps and complete each one you committed to practice today.

- Remember weight in pounds divided by two is the amount in ounces of water you need. You'll know you're hydrated when your urine is clear.

DAY 4

Water is Life-Giving

Remember Mark? What Mark learned was the importance of water even in a healthy person.

I've spent nearly 25 years of my life working in hospitals as a physician. More than 70% of patients that presented with life-threatening trauma need some degree of hydration. Seems very few people drink enough water.

On day two of this week's study, I told you how I answered the question I often receive: "Dr. Marcum, what's the one thing I can do to improve my heart health *today*?"

After I determine if that "one thing" needs to stop tobacco and/or alcohol consumption, I explain that the one thing they can do to improve health immediately is to make sure they're drinking enough pure, fresh water every day. It benefits every single cell in the body.

We studied the first reason why I start with water. Every cell needs water to function correctly and clean our bodies from contaminants inside and out. Water's cleansing properties are a natural truth that God uses to teach us a spiritual truth. We need to be cleansed—first by being saved from the disease of sin inhabiting our very DNA, and secondly we need the daily cleansing from the choices we make that are contrary to God's loving plan. These choices put stress on the body and hurt our relationship with the Ultimate Physician.

Today, we'll focus on another reason why I begin with water.

We simply cannot live without it!

1. **We've already learned that our bodies are composed of 60-70% water**. It's true—God made us to contain water!

2. **Water is necessary in cellular structure, growth, repair and replacement.** In the daily operation of each of our billions of cells, water does everything from providing the internal pressure to keep our cells from collapsing, to providing the fluid medium through which all of the cellular activity moves. The chemical reactions involved in life depend on water. Our cells don't operate in a vacuum. They're filled with water-based fluid that sustains the living environment for all microbiological activity.

So what do these truths about hydration teach us about our spiritual condition? Thankfully, God uses something we understand from our physical experience—water—to explain a spiritual reality.

Read the following passages and mark:

- "water" and its synonyms with a blue oval

- "(God's) Spirit" and His pronouns with a triangle

As a deer pants for flowing streams, so pants my soul for you, O God. My soul thirsts for God, for the living God. (Psalm 42:1,2)

O God, You are my God; earnestly I seek You; my soul thirsts for You; my flesh faints for You, as in a dry and weary land where there is no water. (Psalm 63:10)

With joy you will draw water from the wells of salvation. (Isaiah 12:3)

For I will pour water on the thirsty land, and streams on the dry ground; I will pour my Spirit upon your offspring, and My blessing on your descendants. (Isaiah 44:3)

Come, everyone who thirsts, come to the waters; and he who has no money, come, buy and eat! Come, buy wine and milk without money and without price. (Isaiah 55:1)

Jesus answered, 'Truly, truly, I say to you, unless one is born of water and the Spirit, he cannot enter the kingdom of God.' (John 3:5)

And he said to me, 'It is done! I am the Alpha and the Omega, the beginning and the end. To the thirsty I will give from the spring of the water of life without payment.' (Revelation 21:6)

The Spirit and the Bride say, 'Come.' And let the one who hears say, 'Come.' And let the one who is thirsty come; let the one who desires take the water of life without price. (Revelation 22:1)

When God wants to make sure we don't miss something vital to our life and joy, He reinforces it through repetition. The fact that you can find repetitions of specific themes throughout all sixty-six books of the Bible is even more evidence that a single author inspired the work written through many different writers across a span of more than 2,000 years. What a supernatural display of His love for us—that He would inspire men to communicate His perfect, loving plan to us in a book we can read for ourselves! He also has given us the antidote for our diseased state and Biblical Prescriptions to improve our daily health. This week we have begun with water.

Make a list from what you saw in the above Bible passages about water and the Spirit.

Water	**The Spirit**

_____ _____

_____ _____

_____ _____

_____ _____

_____ _____

Record your answers to these questions.

- In what benefits and functions are they similar? _____

- What is God telling you right now about His Spirit? _____

- What is the value (the worth) of the water that God offers to us? _____

What payment does he require from us to get Living Water?

- Are we putting stress on our brain activating the stress chemistry when we don't take in Living Water? _____

- Do even our genetics long for Spiritual Water? _____

- How much do we have to pay for the Spiritual Water? _____

- In what ways does a gift like this mean we're special and loved very much? _____

WRAPPING IT UP

Can you think of anything that's too valuable to have a price? How about the life of your parent? The life of your child? What about your health? These are examples of things that are so valuable we call them "invaluable," or "unable to be adequately valued."

In God's word, He has shown us something ultimately invaluable—infinitely full of worth and value to the point we can't discuss it in terms of money. There's no amount of money, no price that would be sufficient enough to exchange for _His Spirit_. His Spirit is _priceless_.

Priceless and yet He offers it to us without cost. That means that He offers Himself to us as a _gift_.

If you are a friend of Jesus and have trusted Him and received Living Water, then the gift of the Holy Spirit living within you, springing up eternal life is yours to enjoy. What a treatment for every cell in your body both for the present and future! We could never buy this gift and give it to ourselves. The Spirit has to be given to us by God!

LIVING IN COMMUNITY

Here's another truth that will fill you with awe and wonder. The Spirit of God that lives within me is the same Spirit of God that lives within you. And that Spirit leads us into harmony together and into "all truth" as He teaches us. He primarily teaches us through His written word the Bible. And He uses people like me who are learning His truths and applying them to our area of service. In my case, I'm investing my life and my career in discovering and teaching ways that God has provided for you and me to be healed and journey toward whole-life wellness.

Jesus told His disciples before He sent the Holy Spirit to them on the Day of Pentecost,

> I still have many things to say to you, but you cannot bear them now. When the Spirit of truth comes, he will guide you into all the truth, for he will not speak on his own authority, but whatever he hears he will speak, and he will declare to you the things that are to come. He will glorify me, for he will take what is mine and declare it to you. All that the Father has is mine; therefore I said that he will take what is mine and declare it to you. (John 16:12-15)

There is much more to learn.

BEING MISSIONAL

God loves us so much that He gives us eternal life. He loves us so much that He gives us Himself to live within us. This is good news—immeasurable good news.

Is there someone you know who would be encouraged to know God extends this offer to them as well? Pray for them and to have the opportunity to share with them and serve them.

God's love is extravagant. It's rich. It's overwhelming. And my prayer is that when people meet those of us who are applying Biblical Prescriptions for Life to our lives, they will experience God's unimaginably generous and unconditional love through us.

COMMITMENT

Pause a moment to:

- Practice your memory verses from weeks one and two.

- Are you thinking about drinking enough water daily? Are you partaking of Living Water?

- Review your daily drink journal.

- Celebrate God's goodness toward you and the small changes you are making.

- Determine if you are struggling with consistency. If so, call your study buddy and discuss simple ways that they can help you adopt these Biblical Prescriptions for Life.

- Review your progress. If you think you're moving too slowly, don't give up. Each day is a new day!

- Remember to journal your drink choices in your daily chart.

- Remind yourself of your other simple action steps and complete each one you committed to practice today.

DAY 5

Water is Transformational

We began this week by looking at two passages in the Old Testament—Psalm 1 and Jeremiah 17—to discover how God describes trusting Him and following His ways. It's like being a tree that's healthy and fruit bearing: even in the face of drought! Just imagine what your life would be like if you could experience more of God and His care for you regardless of your circumstances. Troubles come to all; they're unavoidable, inescapable. This means it's not the absence of difficulties but rather the ability to thrive in the midst of them that tells the true story of our health.

This week we've focused on the importance of drinking water to improve our physical health, which in turn improves our spiritual health. Water eases stress on a system. Drinking water is so important. I recently read about research on the dangers of drinking sugary beverages.

Tufts University has studied sweet drinks and concluded that 184,000 deaths (25,000 in the U.S. alone) were tied to these sugary beverages. With these sweet drinks come extra weight and the associated health problems. Researchers analyzed dietary surveys from more than 600,000 people from 51 countries between 1980 and 2010. This was no easy task. They concluded that these fatalities could be in part attributed to sugar-sweetened drinks including sugar-enhanced fruit drinks, sodas, iced teas, and sports drinks—beverages that deliver 50 calories or more per eight-ounce serving.

When I tell people that we all need to drink more liquid, I'm not talking sweet drinks. We need *water* to stay alive and to sustain our body functions. And we need the Living Water to keep us alive spiritually. Both are Biblical Prescriptions that change our chemistry for the good.

Seeking and having access to fresh, clean drinking water is essential and will let us live optimally. Spiritual water will help us through the droughts of life. Write down a few times when you, or someone you love, have experienced a drought. _____

_____

Today, we learn from God's Word how having to access fresh, clean drinking water is physically sustaining. We'll also examine the spiritual corollary: how having God place a source of Living Water within us is eternally sustaining.

Let's read a remarkable interaction recorded for us in the Gospel of John chapter four beginning in verse five.

> So [Jesus] came to a town of Samaria called Sychar, near the field that Jacob had given to his son Joseph. Jacob's well was there; so Jesus, wearied as he was from his journey, was sitting beside the well. It was about the sixth hour.
>
> A woman from Samaria came to draw water. Jesus said to her, "Give me a drink." (For his disciples had gone away into the city to buy food.) The Samaritan woman said to him, "How is it that you, a Jew, ask for a drink from me, a woman of Samaria?" (For Jews have no dealings with Samaritans.) Jesus answered her, "If you knew the gift of God, and whom it is that is saying to you, 'Give me a drink,' you would have asked him, and he would have given you living water." The woman said to him, "Sir, you have nothing to draw water with, and the well is deep. Where do you get that living water? Are you greater than our father Jacob? He gave us the well and drank from it himself, as did his sons and his livestock."
>
> Jesus said to her, "Everyone who drinks of this water will be thirsty again, but whoever drinks of the water that I will give him will never be thirsty again. The water that I will give him will become in him a spring of water welling up to eternal life." The woman said to him, "Sir, give me this water, so that I will not be thirsty or have to come here to draw water" (John 4:5-15).

Here's another geographical reality that demonstrates the reliability of the Bible. The "Jacob" referred to in this story is the patriarch Jacob from the book of Genesis. He's the man who God later renamed Israel. As a travelling shepherd, Jacob and his men dug wells across what is now called "The Holy Land" in order to find water for their flocks. In Jesus' time, many of those wells were still operational. This Samaritan woman used one of Jacob's wells as her family's water source!

- In the passage above, draw a circle around every reference to water.

- What is this passage about? What does the woman know she needs? _____

- What does Jesus know she needs—you may be able to list more than one thing. _____

- Make a list of what we can learn from this passage concerning the two kinds of water the writer John mentions.

The Water from the Well	The Water from Jesus
_____	_____
_____	_____
_____	_____
_____	_____
_____	_____

- What is Jesus telling her about what He alone can give her? _____

- What will she experience if she receives His offer? _____

Do you have this essential in your life? Is it flowing out of your heart? If you don't, ask Jesus for it right now through prayer. It can be as simple as telling Him, "Jesus, I have no life in and of myself. I want to live with You living in and through me. Please send Your Holy Spirit—the Living Water—to live and flow through me."

WRAPPING IT UP

Physical water is essential to life. You won't last longer than a week without it before succumbing to dehydration. The same is true of God's Living Water flowing through you. Though we can live our entire mortal lives without it, we'll never know true, lasting joy without this Living Water coming to our hearts and flowing through us, nourishing our thoughts, will and actions. This Living Water fits us for eternal life.

Seeking Jesus for our daily Living Water—the nourishment only He can give—is an essential Biblical Prescription for Life.

LIVING IN COMMUNITY

Have you started setting a regular time to contact your study buddy and others from your small group? Why not make it a point to pray for people as you read through your small group's list of names. Write down ideas on how you can serve them. As God "the Living Water" leads, call or text them. It's so simple and so very, very powerful. This meaningful way of living together is a Biblical Prescription for Life!

BEING MISSIONAL

The Samaritan Woman becomes the first recorded missionary in the New Testament. Listen to what she does when she returns to her village: "So the woman left her water jar and went away into town and said to the people, 'Come, see a man who told me all that I ever did. Can this be the Christ?' They went out of the town and were coming to him ... Many Samaritans from that town believed in him because of the woman's testimony, 'He told me all that I ever did'" (John 4:28-30, 39)

As you experience changes from following *Biblical Prescriptions for Life*, you will become equipped to go and tell others about what God can do. You won't need to say anything fancy, elaborate, or theologically complex. Just share what He is doing in your life and introduce them to Jesus Himself through the Gospel of John. You can even invite them to join you for your next Biblical Prescriptions for Life small group!

If you can think of someone to invite, write his or her name here now. _____

COMMITMENT

How are you doing practicing and implementing the simple Biblical Prescriptions for Life? So far we've focused on the relationship and drinking water and building good health. If you're not drinking as much water as you know you should, don't give up! Just enjoy a quantity you can drink consistently while increasing, little by little, your net intake. Our goal is to turn down the stress chemistry we learned about in the first week.

Don't judge yourself or others in your group. God grants us success as we make small steps forward on this journey. Most of us move one step at a time to our destinations, usually not with a single superhero-type leap. But we'll get there. Count on it.

DAY 6

The Waters Within Us

Together we've discovered the importance of Living Water—nourishment only God can provide. What's even more astonishing is that He wants to live inside of each one of us. What an honor!

We've learned that God sometimes repeats Himself to make a point. He invites the Samaritan woman to ask Him for Living Water in the Gospel of John chapter four. To make it perfectly clear that invitation is for everyone—even to us today—Jesus extends the invitation to everyone who could hear Him.

Read with me from John chapter seven starting in verse 37: "On the last day of the feast, the great day, Jesus stood up and cried out, 'If anyone thirsts, let him come to me and drink. Whoever believes in me, as the Scripture has said, "Out of his heart will flow rivers of living water."' Now this he said about the Spirit, whom those who believed in him were to receive, for as yet the Spirit had not been given, because Jesus was not yet glorified" (John 7:37-39).

How do we get the Living Water inside of us? Let's remember one of the secrets to healing we learned in our first week together: *God wants us to be willing participants in our healing and journey toward whole-life wellness.*

Stunning, isn't it?

But why? If He has the power to do anything and everything, why does He want us to willingly participate? Consider the sequence of these next statements carefully.

- Coming to God and asking Him for what He offers demonstrates *trust*.

- Trust motivates us to choose His way for our life.

- Making a choice for God based on His character and His promises sets the foundation for a lifetime of *worship*.

We are choosing to accept the gift. As we change and improve our brains through worship, our beliefs change and we begin to make new choices every day--even in the little, seemingly insignificant decisions we make. We are, moment-by-moment, offering our God a *living worship*. I think that's a great way to live and be healthy!

Remember, God never tells us that we need to go out and find Living Water. He sought out the woman at the well and offered it to her. He stood in the crowded center of Jerusalem and offered it to *anyone* who would come. And never does He tell us how we can *earn* Living Water. In fact, He makes it clear that His Living Water is so valuable, it's priceless. It's can't be bought! "And he said to me, 'It is done! I am the Alpha and the Omega, the beginning and the end. To the thirsty I will give from the spring of the water of life without payment'" (Revelation 21:6).

Jesus is offering Living Water to us today. Do you want it? Do you believe He will give it to you if you ask? Do you believe He will give it to you without making you pay for it? If we take Jesus at His word, our job is to simply come to Him and ask Him for it. Then we rest in His arms, trusting that He will provide the Living Water for which our souls desperately thirst.

WRAPPING IT UP

This week we've learned many important things about water—both the physical and spiritual kind. Replacing unhealthy beverage choices with pure fresh water is a Biblical Prescription for Life. Focusing on God's word through Bible reading and memorization is a Biblical Prescription for Life. Both change our physiology and move us away from stress chemistry, which damages the body, and toward the chemistry of love that heals the body.

I'm so glad you've continued on this journey with your small group. It's my prayer that God will bring you healing and so much more as you follow His perfect plan for your life.

LIVING IN COMMUNITY

Don't miss the joy of living—and resting in God's grace—in your special community. We were made for meaningful relationships. They're a Biblical Prescription for Life!

BEING MISSIONAL

Since the first week of study, I've encouraged you to keep a list of one or more names of people who need to experience true inside-out healing. Today might be a good day to call one of them and ask them to spend some time with you tomorrow. You might meet at your place of worship or somewhere peaceful during the day. As the Living Water within you leads, share with them what He is teaching you through *Biblical Prescriptions for Life.*

COMMITMENT

It's time to review your drink journal and the Biblical Prescriptions for Life that you put into practice this week. With what you've learned, transfer the ones you want to adopt for the rest of this study to the master Biblical Prescriptions for Life list at the front of the book now.

DAY 7

Your Day of Rest

Use this space to record notes about today's rest

What spiritual gift did God give you? _____

Where did you rest? _____

Did you join others in their rest? _____

Did you serve someone in an act of selfless love? _____

What did you learn about God today? _____

What did you learn about yourself today? _____

Did the people you have been praying for come to your mind spontaneously? Did you pray for them again?

_____

Did you spend time with anyone from your missional list? What was the result of your time together? Was it what you hoped it would be? _____

A patient went to the doctor's office with many problems. He was surprised that, when he walked through the door, he was warmly welcomed and astonished that there was no paper work or co-pay to wade through. Everyone was smiling and seemed genuinely glad to see him.

The receptionist said that the doctor was standing by to see him *right now*. No waiting. No paperwork. No fee. This was all new to him.

When he went back to the examining room, the doctor listened to his many problems, never once interrupting him! The doctor made him comfortable. Then, the doctor examined him and gave him two prescriptions. The patient was sure he could be successful in these two treatments. Everyone said good- bye and wished him well and out he went. Amazing!

Unfortunately, the patient didn't follow the prescriptions and lapsed back into his old habits and condition. The terrible symptoms returned. He knew he needed help. Sheepishly, he made his way back to the doctor's office in worse condition than before. He was sure that, this time, his welcome would be less than cordial.

But, again, he was warmly welcomed at the office. Everyone was glad to see him. There was no paperwork, co-pay, or wait. The doctor was waiting and once again listened carefully and then offered a treatment plan. The physician reminded the patient that he could come as often as he wanted and he would always be there to welcome

61

and help him. As before, he encouraged the man to start slow with the basics of his treatment. Then, with a warm smile and firm handshake, sent him on his way.

You and I have a Physician who is so much more than this. I don't have words to describe Him. He's always there, always on call, standing by, ready to help us with the symptoms of life and give treatment for the diseases we have. This is the Great Physician we need to come to first for healing. He has told us in His Word, "Come and I will give you rest. I know the rest you need and I will give good gifts to those I love so much" (Matthew 11:28, Luke 11:13).

Rest well and we'll get together again next week.

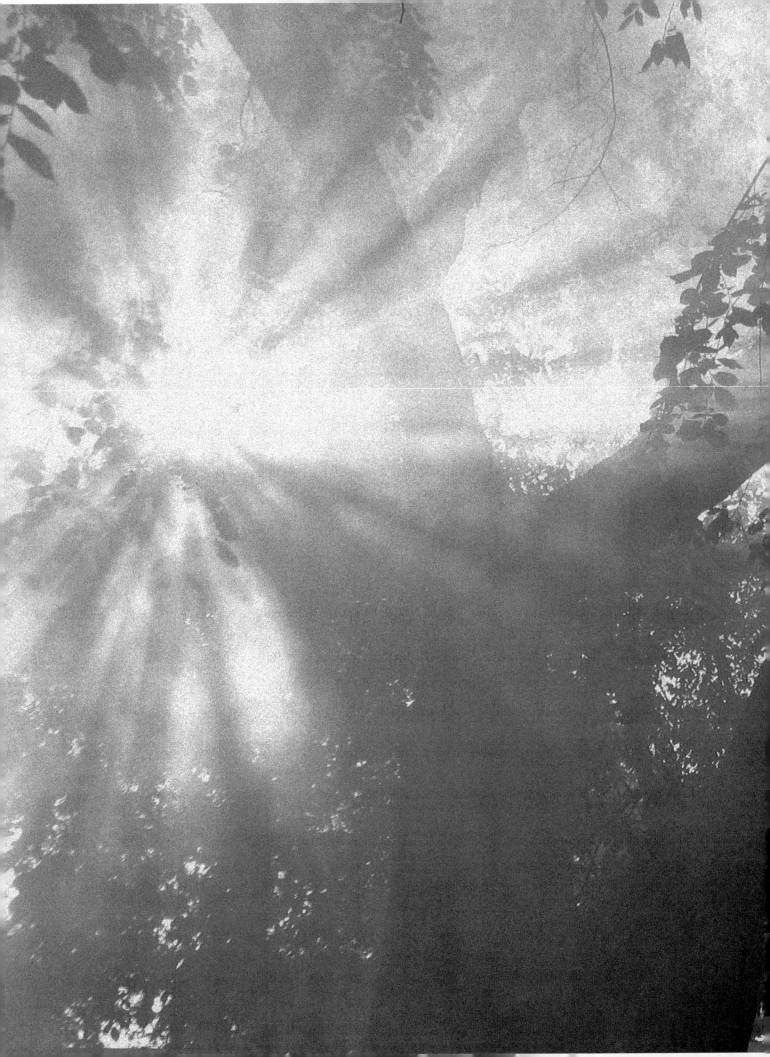

WEEK 3

Biblical Prescription for Life 2—Light for Your Body, Light for Your Soul

Three weeks after the birth of her fourth child, Sarah came in for a follow-up visit. She had a history of an abnormal heart rhythm, which we had successfully surgically ablated. Now her heart was doing fine, but I could tell something was wrong. She wasn't herself. The fourth child had been a surprise to my forty-year-old patient.

After talking to Sarah's, I realized she was depressed. All the symptoms were there—not sleeping, no energy, not happy, not eating, no interest, and very pessimistic. She was living in darkness: not the Sarah I knew.

As she listened, I reviewed the chemistry of depression and how the brain changes. I asked her if she was going outside. She was not. I explained how the sun was needed for Vitamin D production. This pro-hormone helps with chemical reactions throughout the body and helps build and maintain bone, cardiovascular, and brain health as well as giving a boost to our immune system. Basically every cell in our body benefits from Vitamin D. In the brain, this pro-hormone helps produce serotonin, an anti-depressant chemical.

I checked, and, sure enough, Sarah›s Vitamin D levels were woefully low. We gave her some Vitamin D supplements and suggested she go outside for a 30-minute walk three times a week.

In a few weeks, she was back to the Sarah I knew. She was literally walking in the light and had learned a new truth and how to apply that truth to her life.

Instead of reaching for a prescription pad, I had reached for a Biblical Prescription for Life. She was spared an expensive and possibly side-effect-causing medication that would've treated the symptom—depression—without addressing the underlying cause—lack of Vitamin D. Unfortunately medications can cause unintended consequences, side effects. These consequences can cause stress on a body.

It's so simple. Our Creator designed us to be outside. The sun is needed for our body to function at its best. This is part of the original design. Without the sun, stress on the body occurs. In Sarah's case, lack of Vitamin D was decreasing her serotonin levels, which are needed to keep her brain functioning optimally.

Plants need the energy from the sun to live and produce oxygen and food for the world. We need the sun for a host of reactions in the body. It's interesting how we are dependent on the plants and sun for survival. So, what is God telling us? He's saying that we need the sun—and so much more—so we can be productive, serve others, and take care of the world. When we try to move away from these gifts, these truths, stress is the result. Sarah was able to avoid a medication and its possible side effects. More importantly, by adopting a simple, scalable, sustainable Biblical Prescription for Life, she was able to address the underlying issue. She was on the journey to healing and whole-life wellness.

Healthy, moderate sun exposure—what practitioners call "phototherapy"—is a Biblical Prescription for Life. And like all of the Biblical Prescriptions for Life, God can use a physical truth to teach us a spiritual lesson. We need light to survive. In Sarah's case, sunlight enabled her to sleep better, have more energy, increased her serotonin levels, and improved her mood.

Think for a moment, how much time are you spending in the sun? We were designed to be outside and not inside.

Sunshine, via the pro-hormone vitamin D, also acts as natural insulin that lowers blood sugar. Vitamin D strengthens the immune system, lowers blood pressure and can increase cardiac output. Vitamin D helps build bones and prevents osteoporosis. Phototherapy is used to draw toxins out of the skin and can help prevent cancer. The cycle of light and dark regulates the rhythms of the body. These circadian rhythms govern the release of chemical transmitters. These complex interactions help our cells to function optimally as well as help us to rest at night. We have now discovered that certain waves of sunlight can penetrate into the internal organs and promote health. There is so much more to learn. God created light.

What is light? Physical light is described as electromagnetic radiation of varying wavelengths. Some light is visible to us; our brain has the ability to discern certain wavelengths, the visible spectrum. Some light has shorter waves, ultraviolet, while longer waves may be termed infrared. These waves of energy can be emitted or absorbed in packets called photons. This is not a physics course, but I want you to realize the complexities of light. Much about light we are still learning. It only makes sense that our source of energy, light from the sun, is important to health.

Yes, light is important physically. This week we'll also focus on the healing aspects of *spiritual* light.

VIDEO GUIDE 3

Your Citizenship in the Kingdom of Light

VIDEO (20 minutes)

Major Bible verses:

- 1 Peter 2:9

- John 8:12

Who is Sarah? What stands out to you about her? Is there anything in her life you relate to?

Age _____

Symptoms_____

Lifestyle_____

Relationships_____

What is the number one concern people have about sun exposure? _____

Does science support this? _____

Exposure to sunlight is responsible for several vital bodily functions. What are their benefits?

Function	Benefits:
_____	_____

_____   _____

_____   _____

_____   _____

_____   _____

_____   _____

What are the guidelines for how much sun exposure we should get each day?_____

What are simple ways you can start your day feeling more alert and energetic?

_____

_____

_____

Are there ways that light deprivation might be affecting your life? _____

We've learned that it's possible to improve our body's chemistry by simply getting enough sun exposure. Go outside and live in the light! From the ideas you heard in the video, what are some ways you can make this purposeful change? _____

What are the _Biblical Prescriptions for Life_ for Week 3

1. _____

2. _____

3. _____

4. _____

5. _____

6. _____

Group Discussion (20 Minutes)

From Dr. Marcum's video, what most impacted you? Why?

- Describe your mood on a sunny day. How does your body feel in the sun?

- How often do you feel depressed?

- When you feel depressed or discouraged, you may be tempted to retreat into a dark, quiet space. What should you do instead and why?

- How can you balance your concerns about overexposure and skin cancer and the science related to our body's need for natural sunlight each day?

- How much time do you spend outdoors in sunlight each day? Each week?

- When was the last time you spent time outdoors deeply enjoying the beauty of creation and thanking God for His creativity? Share that experience and how it helped you mentally and physically.

With your group, finish this sentence—"*I want to change_____*"

LIVING IN COMMUNITY

We're three weeks into our study of *Biblical Prescriptions for Life*. How are your relationships changing with the people in your small group? Do you see the benefits of investing in these friendships through identifying something simple you can do to purposefully connect with someone in your group each day?

It can be as simple as a text or phone call. I recently traded in my old, low-tech phone and now can even give audio messages! Technology is unbelievable. How about arranging a meet-up for a walk. These encounters help us grow as we communicate honestly with one another.

Almost everyone has some level of concern about sun exposure. For many of us, our beliefs are like pendulums that swing between two extreme positions instead of settling into the midrange of moderation. Maybe this week is a good week to arrange a walk with your study buddy to talk about the ways that you have replaced extreme thoughts with moderate, truth-based thinking that helps you maintain balance and live wisely.

Take time to ask your study buddy or other members of your small group how you can serve them this week as they integrate this Biblical Prescription for Life.

Name	The Best Way I Can Care for Them	Mobile Number

INDIVIDUAL REFLECTION

As you're listened and learned from each other, what is your top-level take-a-way lesson from this week's time together? This is just for you. Write it here. _____

BEING MISSIONAL

Do you know someone who seems to live with a dark cloud over his/her head? They're depressed. Maybe they've sunk into despair. Write their name here and contact them tomorrow. Ask them to get outside with you if even for a 15-minute walk. It will give you both a chance to catch up. And pray that God will use *you* as light in their life even as you help get them out into some healthy sunlight this week.

COMMITMENT

"This week, I am going to ADD and DO at least one of the following simple Biblical Prescriptions for Life:"

I commit to	My Biblical Prescription for Life	Day 1	2	3	4	5	6	7
	Read aloud 5x each day. Practice, memorize & recite:							
	1 John 1:9 *"If we confess our sins, he is faithful and just to forgive us our sins and to cleanse us from all unrighteousness."*							
	John 8:12 *"Again, Jesus spoke to them, saying 'I am the Light of the world. Whoever follows me will not walk in darkness, but will have the light of life.'"*							
	1 Peter 2:9 *"But you are a chosen race, a royal priesthood, a people for his own possession, that you may proclaim the excellencies of Him who called you out of darkness into His marvelous light."*							
	Set your morning alarm and wake up at the same time each day. Start your day with your memory verses in a well-lighted room or with the sunrise in a place you can experience it.							
	Go outside for 15 minutes of sunlight today.							
	While outside, take some moments to be thankful—appreciate God (worship) while outside.							
	Stop using all electronic devices 60 minutes before bed and finish day by reading from a print Bible or encouraging book.							

If you missed a session or want to review one, go to biblicalprescriptionsforlife.com to stream Dr. Marcum's audio and video.

WEEK 3

Ed was thirty-nine and physically dying. A cancer, Non-Hodgkin's' lymphoma, had invaded his body. The irony was that Ed was a fine physician, a friend, and he'd received everything modern medicine had to offer. Nothing worked. Treatment after treatment failed.

I remembered the nights we were on call. He was always the first one to offer an encouraging word, to serve, to help. Now he needed my help.

As the weeks progressed, Ed became weaker physically, but stronger mentally. The chemotherapy was tough; the transfusions and hospitalizations many but Ed continued to get stronger of mind and shared his strength.

I visited him and, at first, the only thing I had to offer was the ministry of presence. As I sat at his bedside, I began to examine my own life. What was I doing? Was I living truth? Was I helping to heal the world? There must be something more to physical well being. Where was truth? Where was meaning? How could Ed be healed?

I'd grown to realize that the Bible was the source of truth and healing. The light prescription, the truth about relationships, so much was found in following Jesus, trusting in Him, believing in Him, and allowing Him—not me— to heal others. Life was so much more than physical health. Healing was more than physical health. Ed understood that the best treatment for his disease—for any disease—was the Light of the Word. He was teaching me this incredible truth.

I hope that during this week together you'll learn not only about how physical light changes our chemistry, but how the spiritual "Light" is needed for ultimate healing. Sometimes, there is nothing we can do physically. We can't earn this healing Light. We must simply believe and accept the treatment. It's a free gift from God.

The Light that physically sustains the world is also the Light Ed had as he dealt with cancer. It's the light we can utilize as we deal with life. Ed would be glad that yet another person is benefitting from his life. My friend, the accomplished physician, had a terminal condition, and yet his life continues to help others heal as I share his story.

DAY 1

As Different as Day and Night

In the healthcare world, we often speak of contrasts. You come to the office because something is not right and it's giving you concern. We call this a symptom. Your heart rhythm might be "atypical" as opposed to normal. The usual "lub-dub" rhythm of blood being forced rhythmically between your heart's atria and ventricles has become another sound with another feeling. You might have blood pressure within the "healthy range" or the "unhealthy range." We might describe someone entering the emergency room as being in "distress" as opposed to enjoying the relative safety you and I are (hopefully) experiencing at this moment.

Understanding contrasts is a very illustrative way of learning. If we know what *typical* is, we can better understand when something is *atypical*.

When God created the universe, He created some very powerful contrasts. He separated the waters at different levels of the atmosphere. He separated the surface of the earth into dry land and oceans and seas. But, the first and foundational contrast He created was the difference between darkness and light.

It's almost impossible to imagine that God began creation without raw materials. But, according to Scripture, there wasn't any dirt, there wasn't any water, there weren't any molecules sitting on some cosmic shelf waiting to be put to work. In fact, there wasn't even "darkness"—He had to create it when He started time!

> In the beginning, God created the heavens and the earth. The earth was without form and void, and darkness was over the face of the deep. And the Spirit of God was hovering over the face of the waters.
>
> And God said, "Let there be light," and there was light. And God saw that the light was good. And God separated the light from the darkness. God called the light Day, and the darkness he called Night. And there was evening and there was morning, the first day. (Genesis 1:1-5)

So, God creates light and darkness on the first day of Creation. On the fourth day, He gives us more detail. We continue at verse 14.

> And God said, "Let there be lights in the expanse of the heavens to separate the day from the night. And let them be for signs and for seasons, and for days and years, and let them be lights in the expanse of the heavens to give light upon the earth." And it was so. And God made the two great lights—the greater light to rule the day and the lesser light to rule the night—and the stars. And God set them in the expanse of the heavens to give light on the earth, to rule over the day and over the night, and to separate the light from the darkness. And God saw that it was good. And there was evening and there was morning, the fourth day. (Genesis 1:14-19)

God creates day and night on the fourth day of creation. Re-read the passages above and circle the words "separate" and "separated."

What did God separate? _____

What are the contrasts? Hint—there are two of them: _____

You might wonder, why didn't God decide to make it daytime all the time? Why separation? Why the contrast?

I know contrasts are very useful in identifying symptoms, diagnosing underlying causes, and determining the best plan of care. It's important to know what is normal and how we were made to function. Then when something is not normal we can quickly identify the change.

As a student of the Bible, I know God can teach us spiritual truths using physical truths. This week, we're going to learn about light. This will change or enhance our core beliefs and propel us to make simple, sustainable, and scalable changes for improving our physical life.

As we study the contrasts God has created, we'll learn another Biblical Prescriptions for Life that can place us on the path to healing and whole-life wellness. We'll again change the chemistry of every cell in our body. Also, in the process of the physical and spiritual development, we'll be changing our DNA and lengthening telomeres as rest and peace replace stress. As we study together, I hope we'll obtain more and more light.

WRAPPING IT UP

If you were seeing me in my office each week over the course of seven weeks, we'd gradually have more and more to talk about. As you started incorporating one or more of each week's Biblical Prescriptions for Life into your new routine, our conversation would inevitably transition to more discussions about why we're making these changes. But, what's even more important to sustaining change is to understand *why* we're following God's Prescriptions for health and wholeness. He's supremely trustworthy. He's motivated by His perfect love for us. And He designed us to live following His good and true plan. He wants us to be healthy.

Have you remembered to drink water? Are you growing in your relationship with the Ultimate Physician? Are you stronger this week than last week? Moving one step at a time is important.

LIVING IN COMMUNITY

We're going to learn very powerful things about physical and spiritual light this week. Two ways you can bring light to someone in your small group today is by calling them and sharing 1. What God is telling you through your memory practice on this week's Bible verses? 2. What are ways that getting outside is benefitting you? Text or call them before the day gets away.

BEING MISSIONAL

I love how God uses light to teach us about Himself and about our need for Him. There's indescribable joy in living in a great relationship with Him. He designed the universe—the darkness, the moon, billions upon billions of stars and even our star, the sun—to reveal Himself to us and show us truths about the unseen spiritual realm. As you learn about light and the life-changing truths about the capital "L" Light, consider people you know at school, work, church or in your community who could use more light in their lives. Then start a conversation!

COMMITMENT

Isn't this rewarding! For many of us, incorporating Biblical Prescriptions for Life starts a whole new process of living, a new lifestyle.

Last week, you selected one or more simple changes from God's teaching that you could apply to your life. Water is vital to health. You documented these changes. If you haven't already done so, transfer those to the pages in the front where you can keep a running *Biblical Prescriptions for Life* plan that lasts throughout the entire course. By the completion of our time together—with God's power and the support of your community—you'll find that you have changed your life in simple, sustainable, and powerful ways. One step at a time you've been growing into wellness. Stay positive!

Our third week offers Biblical Prescriptions for Life to add to your discipline from weeks one and two. I recommend working on this week's actions here and the previous weeks' on page 43. That way you can adjust it if you want to try different ones during the week and move the ones you want to integrate for the long term onto page vii.

Remember:

- Try to get out into the sunlight for 10-15 minutes a day.

- The safest time is before 10 am and after 3 pm.

- Expose your face and body, building to 30 minutes a day.

- If you're turning red, you've been out too long. Cut back.

- If you just cannot get outside, consider a Vitamin D supplement.

- Also we were created to rest when the earth is dark and work when the earth is in light.

The key to sustaining change is integrating simple, scalable actions one step at a time, into your daily routine and accomplishing them within the context of an encouraging, non-judgmental community. Year after year, the patients I've seen succeed with real change and move forward on the path to healing and lifelong whole-life wellness are those who follow this concept. The Biblical Prescriptions for Life God has given us work. But, we have to put them into action. Contrasts help us learn.

DAY 2

God is Where the Light Is

I'm thrilled you're moving forward in this life-changing study of *Biblical Prescriptions for Life*! Feel free to share this knowledge with your friends and family.

With the simple changes we've learned and put in place from weeks one and two, you're probably already noticing a difference in the way you think and feel. I hope you're keeping track of your biometrics as we proceed. I want you to be greatly encouraged by enjoying the changes you are feeling. This is evidence that God is moving in your life.

Yesterday, we learned that God was very deliberate in creating unmistakable contrasts when He formed the universe. One of the most startling contrasts was between *darkness* and *light*.

It's important to remember that God not only created the material universe, He also created the immaterial universe: the rules, logic, and processes that define existence. He created gravity. He created reason. And He created objective truth.

As we've already discovered in weeks one and two, God created the realities of the physical realm and its processes to teach us the realities of the spiritual realm. Keeping this in mind, let's look more closely at the physical distinctions between darkness and light.

- Light is energy.
- The sun gives our earthlight.
- Light is needed by plants for photosynthesis and to make oxygen to breathe and food to eat.
- Light dispels darkness.
- Darkness is the absence of light.
- Light is required for the human eye to see.
- The physical world is visible at varying levels of brightness.
- A point of light can exist in an otherwise dark vacuum, but the converse isn't true.
- Light, in the proper amounts and for the proper duration, can kill bacteria and viruses.
- Light helps activate Vitamin D, a pro-hormone vital for a well-functioning body.
- Light helps regulate our sleep patterns.
- Light helps regulate our stress hormones via circadian rhythms.
- Light is involved in other bodily reactions we have yet to discover.

Looking at that list, it's evident that light makes things visible and is needed for our well being. Light and darkness do not co-exist well. In fact, darkness cannot smother light. Light must be extinguished or covered for darkness to prevail.

We've already seen how God can use physical reality to teach us about spiritual reality—using a concept we understand to teach us one that may be more difficult to grasp. He's revealing a realm—the spiritual reality—that many of us have never known or emphasized. Some have even chosen to ignore that realm.

God made light in the first day of creation. Then He made day and night—and the lights that govern them—on the fourth day of creation. He did this perhaps to create distinctions—separations—between darkness and light in the world; separations so fundamental to our existence that we couldn't possibly ignore them, explain them away, or fail to orient our very lives around them.

Knowing this, what is the Great Physician trying to teach us about light and darkness in the spiritual reality? "Darkness" is used in the Bible to describe literal absence of physical light (in clouds, at night). What mankind has added is other another use of *darkness*, namely the active avoidance of God to commit selfish, harmful acts against other people (Ephesians 5:11). In fact, the contrast doctrine of "darkness" is a significant, cautionary theme running throughout the Bible.

As we work diligently to reprogram our neural pathways through simple Biblical Prescriptions for Life, today we're going to focus on LIGHT as made evident by Truth, God's character, His presence, and by love. Let's train our minds to think about Him and the wholeness that comes from living in a right relationship with Him.

Read carefully through the following passages and circle every reference to light—and anything bright and glowing (i.e., "light", "radiance", "shine", "glow", "(burning) fire", "brightness", etc. and their synonyms).

> (Ezekiel is describing his vision of God) And upward from what had the appearance of his waist I saw as it were gleaming metal, like the appearance of fire enclosed all around. And downward from what had the appearance of his waist I saw as it were the appearance of fire, and there was brightness around him. Like the appearance of the bow that is in the cloud on the day of rain, so was the appearance of the brightness all around. (Ezekiel 1:27-28)

> Out of Zion, the perfection of beauty, God has shone forth. (Psalm 50:2)

> And behold, the glory of the God of Israel was coming from the way of the east and His voice was like the sound of many waters; and the earth shone with His glory. (Ezekiel 43:2)

> And an angel of the Lord suddenly stood before them, and the glory of the Lord shone around them; and they were terribly frightened. (Luke 2:9)

> Then the glory of the LORD went up from the cherub to the threshold of the temple, and the temple was filled with the cloud and the court was filled with the brightness of the glory of the LORD. (Ezekiel 10:4)

> (Matthew is describing Jesus after He had risen from the grave) And his appearance was like lightning, and his clothing as white as snow. (Matthew 28:3)

> ... to keep the commandment unstained and free from reproach until the appearing of our Lord Jesus Christ, which he will display at the proper time—he who is the blessed and only Sovereign, the King of kings and Lord of lords, who alone has immortality, who dwells in unapproachable light, whom no one has ever seen. (1 Timothy 6:14, 15)

> After these things I saw another angel coming down from heaven, having great authority, and the earth was illumined with his glory. (Revelation 18:1)

The word describing, "Light" and its synonyms	What the word is describing for us
_____	_____
_____	_____
_____	_____
_____	_____
_____	_____
_____	_____
_____	_____

Making a list like this is important for several reasons. First, when I'm studying something I need to learn, I have to slow down and be methodical about what the text says. You have no choice but to slow down when you mark key words. Secondly, recording important details of the topic helps me learn and retain what the author is trying to communicate. Making a list is a powerful way to get the significant points out of any passage about a key concept.

So you have your list—good work! Now, most importantly, what is God telling *you* about Himself through your study of light as it refers to His presence? _____

Does this description of God's character—His perfect purity—give you a desire to know Him more and why?

_____

Record any additional thoughts before we conclude today's study.

_____

WRAPPING IT UP

What 's the most beautiful "thing" you can think of? Try to describe it. You can use many words and still not feel like you've done it justice. How do you distill the essence of that person, place or thing into just one or two words?

As you've gone outside in the sunlight today, how did the warmth of the sun feel to you? Think about all the chemistry the sunlight is turning on. Your belief that God is using the power of the sun in your healing will enhance the effect.

For our God—the Creator of the heavens and earth—one of most powerful ways to describe His essence is *light*; pure, perfect, unadulterated (that just means "unmixed"), vision-enabling, truth revealing, clean *light*. There is nothing like it. There's nothing like God.

Thankfully, He has given us other one-word descriptors for Himself. We'll learn about a very special one of those in day five this week. It's my prayer that you can feel God's perfect, revealing light shining on you today.

LIVING IN COMMUNITY

Did your study buddy learn something about God today that he/she never knew before? Find out! Just asking the question will draw meaningful conversation out and help grow a real relationship between the two of you. Remember, relationships are a Biblical Prescription for Life!

BEING MISSIONAL

Many of us love light. If you know someone who seems to be overwhelmed by darkness, take time right now to pray for him or her. You might even ask God to reveal Himself to them, to remove the darkness with His pure, perfect, life-giving light. How about inviting someone like that to join you outside to walk or sit in the sunshine?

COMMITMENT

Take a look at your *Biblical Prescriptions for Life* commitments from week one through this week. Are you keeping the simple actions from the first two weeks as you move into week three? If not, don't be critical or get down on yourself. Maybe you just need to move slowly. If you want to—no matter what yesterday was like—you can start again today. Try to get outside every day and write down the time you spend outdoors. Make this an important activity just like drinking water or brushing your teeth. Also work on resting at night and not staying up too late. This will help your light-mediated rhythms. Keep in mind that for us to have light, we need to be with God.

DAY 3

You Can't Bring a Pinpoint of Darkness into a Room full of Light

Yesterday was a significant day of learning for us. I know this is true because whenever we spend time with God (worship), we've done something that changes our beliefs for our ultimate benefit. Those changes create a cascade of adjustments to our actions—beliefs drive actions—and even alter our body's chemistry.

Thus, the premise of *Biblical Prescriptions for Life*:

Knowing God changes us. Being in a relationship with Him brings us wholeness. Reorienting our lives to follow His original design for us reduces stress and puts in place the path to healing and life-long, whole-life wellness.

We studied about God and His presence yesterday. There can be no more significant topic for us to study. As I just said, knowing Him is the very basis for health.

So, let's start today's time together by remembering what we learned concerning God's presence. Our "presence" is what it's like for someone else to experience our personhood. It would be very valuable to summarize key truths about God as they relate to light.

- Light is **purity of character**—no selfishness, no wavering from consistent goodness, no un-lovingness at all.

- Light is **truth**—no error, no deception, no partial understanding

- God is so true, so pure, so incomparably good and whole, that **He Himself dwells in inapproachable light.** *Inapproachable.* It's so bright, so pure, so unfiltered that darkness cannot even get near. His enemy the devil—who dwells in darkness and does his harmful work in darkness—can't approach Him.

So, this is today's big idea as we adopt this light-related Biblical Prescription for Life. Even though it's a very humbling truth, I want you to stay with me.

God is light and dwells in inapproachable light. We simply can't approach him in our current condition.

But here's the dilemma: light is also life-giving. We observe this in our physical world. Light is energy. We've already seen how our body craves light for important reactions. Without it, every cell is stressed. Technology has taught us about Vitamin D, the importance of plant energy, and the regulation of stress chemicals via circadian rhythms. There's more that technology hasn't uncovered. Light is our energy source, our power source. Think about it. How would you feel without an energy source? How does your car run without gasoline in the tank? As we continue to learn about light, I want you to begin to feel empowered because there's a source of energy on reserve for those who know where to find it!

Being separated from God—the Light of the World—is not good news. We were designed for this relationship, which provides an open channel to this light, this energy. Without this spiritual light illuminating our lives, our bodies become stressed. We're missing much more than Vitamin D, strong bones, and circadian rhythms.

We'll learn about the good news, the path to God and his marvelous light, tomorrow.

In week one, we learned that, thanks to Adam, we have selfishness—the opposite of love, what the Bible calls *sin*—in our very DNA. Because of this inherited contamination, and because of the choices we have made, we're no longer in the original, pure, untainted condition in which God created us. We now have "darkness" inside us. Truth be told, sometimes we feel more comfortable in darkness, especially when we're intent on a selfish pursuit.

When we choose selfishness, we downshift our brain away from relationships that serve and love. We focus, instead, on the attitudes and actions that create stress. All of this takes place in the lower part of our brain where we generate our infamous "fight or flight" response. That response is concerned about staying alive. It focuses on "looking out for number one"! This response—when placed in the "on" position for great lengths of time, can turn on the stress chemistry and literally change our brains. We become selfish. It's all about me. I must preserve "myself." It's a reflex we share with reptiles!

Read the following passages and mark every occurrence of the word "darkness" and its synonyms with a rectangle.

> And this is the judgment: the light has come into the world, and people loved the darkness rather than the light because their works were evil. For everyone who does wicked things hates the light and does not come to the light, lest his works should be exposed. But whoever does what is true comes to the light, so that it may be clearly seen that his works have been carried out in God. (John 3:19-20)
>
> For the wrath of God is revealed from heaven against all ungodliness and unrighteousness of men, who by their unrighteousness suppress the truth. For what can be known about God is plain to them, because God has shown it to them. For his invisible attributes, namely, his eternal power and divine nature have been clearly perceived, ever since the creation of the world, in the things that have been made. So they are without excuse. For although they knew God, they did not honor him as God or give thanks to him, but they became futile in their thinking, and their foolish hearts were darkened. Claiming to be wise, they became fools, and exchanged the glory of the immortal God for images resembling mortal man and birds and animals and creeping things. (Romans 1:18-23)

I don't like spending time making a list of very negative things. I find that sharing the risks associated with lifestyle choices help my patients make good decisions. Believe it or not, some do not even realize the risks of their choices. Consequences reveal truth. As we've seen about the Creation account, these distinctions and separations are instructive. They are ultimately for our good if they point us away from stress and toward a right relationship with our Creator.

Try to correlate the above verses with the human condition.

The word describing "darkness" and its synonyms	what that word is describing for us
_____	_____
_____	_____
_____	_____

Why did people who are made in God's image choose darkness?

In John chapter 3? _____

In Romans chapter 1? _____

It's very clear that there's an eternally significant purpose in the distinctions God has made between darkness and light. He has created a world where this distinction is physically unavoidable. And according to His words found in the Bible, it's equally unavoidable in the unseen spiritual reality.

Let's stop now and ask Him to help us make sense of this very significant concept. We can just talk to Him. Something like:

> *"Father, because you love me, you have shown truths to me for my good and for my wellness. I struggle to fully understand what you're showing me. I am even struggling right now with the very sad idea of people being separated from you. But I trust that you are light and love and that you have made a way for us to be in a right relationship with you no matter how dark our world has been. Amen."*

WRAPPING IT UP

Depression is often described in terms of darkness. So is addiction. In these darkened conditions, we'll stay in darkness unless God Himself intervenes. I encouraged you to get to the fourth day of this week's study where we'll learn that God Himself has provided a way for us to return to the Kingdom of Light and to remain there even when we temporarily fall back to our old ways of thinking and harmful habits.

LIVING IN COMMUNITY

Review the names of the people in your small group, starting with your study buddy. Look at the areas in which they've expressed a desire for change. Think about the notes you've made about ways you can support them. God loves them like He loves you. Pray for them, that they can experience God's love in a very real way today. Then reach out to one or two and let them know that you care about them and prayed for them specifically. The ministry of presence is a ministry of service.

BEING MISSIONAL

We live in a world that's under temporary management. God created it "good, very good" but mankind's first parents traded God's ways for their own. Because our ancestors Adam and Eve chose to live by their own rules, darkness is the default condition of our understanding. As God is revealing Himself and His ways to you through *Biblical Prescriptions for Life*, continue to pray for the person you identified yesterday. And be ready for the opportunity to share the light of God with them when it presents itself.

COMMITMENT

Of the simple, Biblical Prescriptions for Life each of us are adopting, the most powerful ones are the deliberate memorization of God's words to us. They create the change in our beliefs that motivate new, healing behaviors. They change our body's chemistry. And they give us the hope to persevere even when we do so imperfectly. Be encouraged today. Focus on God. Give thanks to Him. And work on your chosen Biblical Prescriptions for Life from week one through week three this day. Also, don't forget to get outside and feel the warmth of light and enjoy the chemical benefits. Try to get to bed a few minutes earlier each evening to improve your circadian rhythms. This will improve your stress chemistry. Take time to thank God right now for the light He gives each day so we can live forever. Is the Creator of physical light the power source in your life? Remember, to approach that light we need Jesus.

DAY 4

Being in the Light makes us Glow

I hope during the course of studying *Biblical Prescriptions for Life* you learn that an encounter with God's Word is an encounter with God. He wrote the Bible for us. He wants us to know Him. He loves us that much!

Spending time with God in His word and trusting Him to lead us into all understanding will change us. I've seen how spending time with God changes my patients from the inside out. These changes have been observed on lab reports, biometrics, on medications needed, and in the general well being of patients. Rest replaces stress. Later this week we'll explore the technology and the evidence-based research that supports God's word.

But for now, let me ask you a question. What does being in light look like? Will others see something different when they look at us?

Moses wanted to know God. He wanted a relationship with Him. In fact, he was willing to risk his life to see God. What was the risk? God is light in such a pure, powerful, holy way, that no man is free of darkness enough to see Him face-to-face and live!

> And the Lord said to Moses, "This very thing that you have spoken I will do, for you have found favor in my sight, and I know you by name." Moses said, "Please show me your glory." And [God] said, "I will make all my goodness pass before you and will proclaim before you my name 'The Lord.' And I will be gracious to whom I will be gracious, and will show mercy on whom I will show mercy. But," he said, "You cannot see my face, for man shall not see me and live." And the Lord said, "Behold, there is a place by me where you shall stand on the rock, and while my glory passes by I will put you in a cleft of the rock, and I will cover you with my hand until I have passed by. Then I will take away my hand, and you shall see my back, but my face shall not be seen. (Exodus 33:17-23)"

Remember—God's presence was the experience of being *near* Him. When the word "glory" is used in the Bible as a noun, it indicates the manifestation of His presence. As we study together, are we near Him?

God knew that none with sin-stained DNA could be in His perfectly pure and radiant presence and survive. He wanted to protect Moses from certain death, like I would protect my children from staring at the sun or from getting too close to a nuclear reaction.

Being in God's presence and beholding His glory (His presence) even from an indirect view—made a very real change in Moses. Let's continue reading:

> When Moses came down from Mount Sinai, with the two tablets of the testimony in his hand as he came down from the mountain, Moses did not know that the skin of his face shone because he had been talking with God. Aaron and all the people of Israel saw Moses, and behold, the skin of his face shone, and they were afraid to come near him. (Exodus 34:29, 30)

Did you catch something very special here? Being with God—listening to Him, even just having God pass by—was being in His inapproachable light! What in these passages makes it very clear that Moses experienced God's pure, perfect, supernaturally powerful light? _____

As you reflect, what is God teaching us this week?

1. God created physical light and darkness. Light is an energy source.

2. Light is needed for the normal function of the body. Lack of light produces stress.

3. God *separated* physical light from physical darkness.

4. Physical light dispels physical darkness; they can't coexist.

From the physical realm, God has designed powerful ways to help us understand the equally real spiritual realm.

1. As we learned with Moses, God dwells in light.

2. In God's presence, there can be no darkness.

3. The light of God's presence has health benefits.

Here's today's supernatural truth: God wants to bring us into His presence, His light, so we can live in an intimate relationship with Him. Let me say this again: *God wants to bring us into His presence so we can live in an intimate relationship with Him.*

Wow! The God of the universe wanting to be my closest friend! The God of the universe wanting to give me real power to live my life. Just like the sun provides physical energy power to each and every plant on earth, God wants to give me—and you, and each and every person on earth—spiritual energy power to serve out our mission of love and care for all creation.

Please pause for a moment to consider those enormous truths.

How does God desire to make you feel? Loved. Valued. Desired. Special.

To bridge the gap between His holiness—the fact that He dwells in pure, perfect, inapproachable light—and our current sinful condition, God must provide a way for us to enter His presence, His light.

Read the following passage and mark:

* "Light" with a star

* "Darkness" with a shaded rectangle

> This is the message we have heard from him and proclaim to you, that God is light, and in him is no darkness at all. If we say we have fellowship with him while we walk in darkness, we lie and do not practice the truth. But if we walk in the light, as he is in the light, we have fellowship with one another, and the blood of Jesus his Son cleanses us from all sin. If we say we have no sin, we deceive ourselves, and the truth is not in us. If we confess our sins, he is faithful and just to forgive us our sins and to cleanse us from all unrighteousness. If we say we have not sinned, we make him a liar, and his word is not in us. (1 John 1:5-10)

Darkness is synonymous with:

_____

_____

_____

_____

Darkness keeps us from:

_____

_____

_____

_____

Light is synonymous with:

_____

_____

_____

_____

Lights allows us to:

_____

_____

_____

_____

Jesus' disciple John (the human writer of First John) gives us two more big connections in this packed passage.

From what do we need to be cleansed? _____

Does everyone have this contaminant and how do we know this? _____

What can we do? _____

This is what Christians call "The Gospel"! The fact is only Jesus can cleanse us from the selfish, stressful contamination that keeps us from God's presence. And just like we need to get outside into daylight every day, God's Word tells us we need to practice the confession of our sins whenever we move into darkness. We need to get into the daylight of a right relationship with God. When we have light, we have healing. Without light, there is darkness.

Confession is agreeing with God that we chose to live according to our plan instead of His; we acted selfishly; we created stress in our bodies and in our relationships. Shouldn't we all humbly pray?

"Father, I chose to (specific thought or action) and go my own way instead of following Your loving plan

for me. I'm sorry. I don't want to walk in darkness. I want to walk in the light with You. Thank You for
loving me. Thank You for being the light that overpowers darkness. Amen."

Once we confess our shortcomings, we're forgiven. Our sins are thrown into "the depths of the sea" (Micah 7:19) and are forgotten. We would do well to learn to do the same.

God also understands that we can't possibly remember all of our shortcomings. It's impossible. So, I often pray a prayer something like this: "God I have sinned. I can't even remember all the times that I have let You down. Thank You for forgiving them all and throwing them away through the gift of your Son. I accept that gift and believe in your Son. Also help me to see where I am living apart from your plan."

WRAPPING IT UP

Have you ever had sun-kissed skin: that gentle glow from being outside and getting just enough sun exposure to warm your skin and your complexion? That's a physical demonstration of a spiritual reality.

When we live in the presence of God, we enjoy the warmth and beautification of being in His light. Like Moses, our very countenances can shine with the radiance of a right relationship with our loving God.

LIVING IN COMMUNITY

There are two very special results of walking in the light with Jesus. You'll find them in 1 John 1:7.

Write them here: _____

That's right—and it's exactly the way God designed it. Being in a right relationship with God allows us to not only be forgiven, but also to enter into right relationships with others. Remember, He designed us for relationship. It's how we experience healing. And when we hurt one another—intentionally or unintentionally—confession and restoration is the path to wholeness and peace. The opposite of stress is rest. You can have peace in your relationships starting today!

BEING MISSIONAL

Have you ever had someone ask you, "What makes you so...different?" Maybe they saw you respond to a harsh person with gentleness. Maybe they saw you give selflessly instead of getting more "stuff" for yourself. Whether you realize it or not, that difference is the glow of God's presence in your life. It may not look like you just returned from a beach vacation, but it is an undeniable radiance that reflects the irresistible goodness of God's pure, perfect light.

Walking in the light shows that we're citizens of the Kingdom of Light.

1 Peter 2.9 - "But you are a chosen race, a royal priesthood, a holy nation, a people for his own possession, that

you may proclaim the excellencies of him who called you out of darkness into His marvelous light.

Loving people is a way to be meaningfully missional everyday. You're being watched. Be ready to tell all who are willing to listen why you love the way you do.

COMMITMENT

I love the memory verses that we have selected in *Biblical Prescriptions for Life*. I encourage you to spend time reciting and meditating on the healing words of 1 John 1:9 today. There we find hope for each of us!

Are you using light to improve your health? Did you go outside today? Are you working on resting more while it is dark to improve the rhythms of life? Light is a Biblical treatment, both physical and spiritual light.

If you have a moment, send me an email. Let me know how this study is going for you. I 'd like to serve you and your study group by praying for you. Also, take a look at yourself in the mirror. I'll bet you're glowing!

DAY 5

How to Walk in the Light of the Son

Yesterday, we discovered the unbelievable kindness of God as we studied His path for leaving darkness and returning to His marvelous light. Walking in the light is evidence of our right relationship with God and people will notice a difference.

Today, let's start by thanking God for forgiving us and for making us citizens of His Kingdom of Light. You don't need special words, just tell Him *"thank you, Father."* Tell Him in your own words.

> *"Father, thank You for sunshine, not only because it's good for my health and provides energy to our planet, but because I'm reminded that You are the Light of the world. Thank You for creating me in Your likeness. Help me to bring light and warmth to those around me."*

God has provided a way back into His presence, a way back to light, a way back to the source of life. It's while living in His presence that we begin to fully understand our selfishness, our darkness, and agree that His way is better for us. We learn to trust Him and His promise to restore our relationship with Him. We actually yearn to be with Him. This light is an energy source for our soul.

Jesus became a human to empathize with our weaknesses. He offers to give us His right standing with God. When God looks at us, He sees Jesus' perfection and love, not the "filthy rags" or our sin. We've been given something we could never earn. It's a gift.

Now, free from our darkness and separation from God, we can be restored to a loving, growing, joyful relationship with the Father. I can honestly tell you that is *the best news* I—or you—can share with anyone. Just as the plants need light to give life, we need Jesus for life. It's His kindness that enables us to avoid dangerous detours into darkness. It's His kindness that shows us the path to joyful living on our journey to healing and life-long, whole-life wellness. He invites us to live in the light!

Are you ready for even more "best news"?

Read these passages and mark:

- Light and its synonyms with a star.

- Darkness and its synonyms with a shaded rectangle.

- Jesus (and His pronouns) with a cross.

- When Jesus refers to Himself as light—draw a star over the cross.

- People who follow Jesus (i.e., "we", "ourselves", "you", etc.) with your name.

Again Jesus spoke to them, saying, "I am the light of the world. Whoever follows me will not walk in darkness, but will have the light of life. (John 8:12)"

This is the message we have heard from him and proclaim to you, that God is light, and in him is no darkness at all. If we say we have fellowship with him while we walk in darkness, we lie and do not practice the truth. But if we walk in the light, as he is in the light, we have fellowship with one another, and the blood of Jesus his Son cleanses us from all sin. If we say we have no sin, we deceive ourselves, and the truth is not in us. If we confess our sins, he is faithful and just to forgive us our sins and to cleanse us from all unrighteousness. If we say we have not sinned, we make him a liar, and his word is not in us. (1 John 1:5-10)

So Jesus said to them, "The light is among you for a little while longer. Walk while you have the light, lest darkness overtake you. The one who walks in the darkness does not know where he is going. While you have the light, believe in the light, that you may become sons of light. (John 12:35, 36)"

Whoever says he is in the light and hates his brother is still in darkness. Whoever loves his brother abides in the light, and in him there is no cause for stumbling. (1 John 2:9, 10)

For you are my lamp, O Lord, and my God lightens my darkness. For by you I can run against a troop, and by my God I can leap over a wall. This God—his way is perfect; the word of the Lord proves true; he is a shield for all those who take refuge in him. (2 Samuel 22:29-31)

And this is the judgment; the light has come into the world, and people loved the darkness rather than the light because their works were evil. For everyone who does wicked things hates the light and does not come to the light, lest his works should be exposed. But whoever does what is true comes to the light, so that it may be clearly seen that his works have been carried out in God. (John 3:19-21)

Besides this you know the time that the hour has come for you to wake from sleep. For salvation is nearer to us now than when we first believed. The night is far gone; the day is at hand. So then let us cast off the works of darkness and put on the armor of light. (Romans 13:11, 12)

Make a list of what you learned simply by marking these key concepts straight from these Bible passages about:

Darkness—What did you learn about darkness and those who live in darkness?

_____

_____

_____

_____

_____

Light—Who is Light? What concepts are described as light?

_____

_____

_____

_____

_____

How can someone put on God's light and even *become* Light?

_____

_____

_____

_____

_____

What are the benefits of being in the light, walking in the light, and living in the light?

_____

_____

_____

_____

_____

How does someone enter and live in the light?

_____

_____

_____

_____

Jesus tells us *how* we can live in the light with Him and others who are following Him. These are Biblical Prescriptions for Life! I'm breathless with gratitude that God desires a relationship with me and has provided the way for me to know Him, please Him, and find my ultimate joy in Him!

Now, read aloud the passages where you replaced the pronouns for followers of Jesus with your name. These are tremendous statements about your identity—who you are and who we are becoming on this journey to whole-life wellness. What is God telling you as you hear these words while you speak them? Write them here before you move on and get distracted.

_____

WRAPPING IT UP

What a GREAT God who made us; so very great that He would create physical light and darkness so that we could understand His character and the spiritual reality that surrounds us unseen. I'm speechless.

What is God saying to you right now? Are you hearing His love for you through His word, the Bible? Are you becoming thankful? Is your desire to continue growing? Mine sure is. And it, love, grows each day I spend time with Him. I can wholeheartedly agree with Christian author A.W. Tozer who wrote, "To have found God and still to pursue Him is the soul's paradox of love, scorned indeed by the too-easily-satisfied religionist, but justified in happy experience by the children of the burning heart."

LIVING IN COMMUNITY

By now, you probably don't even need to refer to your list of fellow students to remember the ways you can support them. And you probably have their phone numbers in your contact list. I encourage you to invest time today in these very special, growing relationships. Maybe there's someone you haven't connected with yet. Today is a great day to try again! There's simply too much astoundingly good news in today's study to keep to yourself. Call and share it. Ask them to share what God is saying to them and doing in their heart.

BEING MISSIONAL

"God loves you and wants to have a great relationship with you. And He provided the way!" What a refreshing truth to share with someone. As we're completing week three of *Biblical Prescriptions for Life*, you've probably made a list of three or four people for whom you've been praying and purposely engaging with God's path to healing and wellness. Pray for them right now. And then plan a time to connect with at least one of them today.

COMMITMENT

Contemplation, memorization, recitation—these are profound tools in rewiring our neural pathways. They are especially necessary when we have specific harmful thoughts to discard and replace with healing thoughts. It takes purpose. It takes practice. And it takes time. Just like small, simple, changes in diet and exercise create life-changing benefits over time, so do changes in our beliefs. That's why reading, meditating, and memorizing Bible truths are a key Biblical Prescription for Life. Also, did you get outside today? Even if it's cold, you still need the physical light.

If you find that you're not yet able to recite verses from weeks one, two, and three by this point, don't be discouraged and don't give up. Write them out on 3x5 cards and put them places where you'll see them frequently throughout the day. I try to start each day by reading and reciting these biblical truths. I try to end each day the same way.

In the first few weeks of *Biblical Prescriptions for Life* we've focused on the importance of relationships, drinking water, and being thankful for sunlight. These prescriptions change our health for the good and affect the entire body. Every cell benefits. God's Prescriptions do not help one organ and hurt another and, like all good gifts from Him, are available to all.

As we are growing in the relationship with God, our brain chemistry and structure is also changing. God creates a new brain with different chemistry as we walk with Him. As we'll soon learn, this change has an effect on the *entire* body. We are moving toward love and away from selfishness, one step at a time.

DAY 6

Night Lights, Sunbeams and Candles in the Dark

When Jesus returned to heaven, He deliberately left His followers behind to continue His work on earth. He could have stopped time or taken all the people who trusted Him to heaven with Him. Instead, His plan was—and continues to be—to depend on "agents of light" who will introduce their families, friends and communities to God in His physical absence. This is our mission, our reason for being.

He designed physical light to shine on our planet: to shine throughout the solar system, throughout the universe, and into our galaxy. Light is the energy source. That's His awesome plan. He wants us to shine spiritual light throughout the universes of our relationships! People notice light in a dark room just as they'll notice hope in a hopeless world. Do you consider yourself a star of spiritual light?

Honestly, I'm thankful for His plan. I wouldn't have known about God's love for me if it hadn't been for my earthly family demonstrating it to me every day of my life.

Remember, God the Father dwells in inapproachable light. We can't enter His presence or live in His light without Jesus' perfection overcoming (or "covering") our imperfection first. Once we become "children of light," we keep our relationship with Him clear by confessing when we have chosen darkness—selfishness, being unloving—over His way of love, His way of light.

Before we dive in today, I want us to read what Paul wrote to the followers of Jesus living in Ephesus.

> Now this I say and testify in the Lord, that you must no longer walk as the Gentiles do, in the futility of their minds. They are darkened in their understanding, alienated from the life of God because of the ignorance that is in them, due to their hardness of heart. (Ephesians 4:17, 18)

What strikes you from these two short verses?

For me, I see that once Jesus has made us a citizen of His Kingdom of light, the lifestyle of living in the light is a choice.

I see the evidence, all around, of people—and whole nations—being outside of a relationship with God. What's happening to our world? Is it a better place? Also, those who choose to live outside of God's *physical* laws, whether it's not drinking enough water or hiding from the sunlight, are having physical problems.

From what we've learned about spiritual darkness—can you list some examples you've seen in relationships around you? Be discerning. Write in terms of the lack of light and the damage it creates, not in terms of speaking critically about any specific person you know. This will help reinforce our study as we look at the evidence around us.

_____

Also, can you list ways where not being in the physical sunlight might harm your physical well-being?

_____

Now, I want you to list some specific examples of ways that you've seen followers of Jesus be a light to you and others you know. It's okay to name names here—just make sure to thank God as you remember the light He has shown through these lights He's placed in your life.

_____

I want to make sure we always leave our minds in the "upshift" mode—the relational, loving, selfless, giving mode.

I want us to focus on the positive. This is a way we can actively participate with God as He rewires our neural pathways and brings healing into our lives. This is His good plan for us—and He built it into each one of us.

Let's briefly review what we've learned this week.

- God is light.

- God dwells in light.

- Jesus covers our failure and replaces our shortcomings with His perfection. This enables us to enter into and continue to live in God's light-saturated presence.

- When we are in His light, there will be noticeable changes.

- Following Jesus is how we walk in the Light.

- Our mission is to share Light.

Now for more good stuff.

Read the following passages and mark:

- Light and its synonyms with a star

- Jesus and His pronouns with a cross

- God the Father with a triangle

- People who follow Jesus (i.e., "we", "ourselves", "you", etc.) with your name

And as a helpful hint, Jesus is speaking in the passages from John chapter 17 and Matthew chapter 5.

> I have manifested your name to the people whom you gave me out of the world. Yours they were, and you gave them to me, and they have kept your word. Now they know that everything that you have given me is from you. For I have given them the words that you gave me, and they have received them and have come to know in truth that I came from you; and they have believed that you sent me. I am praying for them. I am not praying for the world but for those whom you have given me, for they are yours. All mine are yours, and yours are mine, and I am glorified in them. And I am no longer in the world, but they are in the world, and I am coming to you. Holy Father, keep them in your name, which you have given me, that they may be one, even as we are one. (John 17:6-11)"

> For God, who said, "Let light shine out of darkness," has shone in our hearts to give the light of the knowledge of the glory of God in the face of Jesus Christ. (2 Corinthians 4:6)

> For it is God who works in you, both to will and to work for his good pleasure. Do all things without grumbling or disputing, that you may be blameless and innocent, children of God without blemish in the midst of a crooked and twisted generation, among whom you shine as lights in the world. (Philippians 2:13-15)

> You are the light of the world. A city set on a hill cannot be hidden. Nor do people light a lamp and put it under a basket, but on a stand, and it gives light to all in the house. In the same way, let your light shine before others, so that they may see your good works and give glory to your Father who is in heaven. (Matthew 5.14-16)

In what ways are we to be light?

_____

_____

_____

_____

_____

There are several reasons why God has designed us to be light to the world around us. What are they?

_____

_____

_____

_____

_____

Our lives become joyful, satisfying, and life-giving as we live as children of light. It's so very good for us to live with God in His presence. Science is just now beginning to document the physiological improvements we experience as we live God's way. Our technology today is not yet advanced enough to capture *all* the physiologic improvements. Scientists are beginning to learn more about the positive chemical and physical changes in our body, especially in the brain—the control center. God has known what was best for us all along. Science now has the technology through PET scans, functional MRI's, and other sophisticated devices to begin to understand the physiology of His creation. But we know the reason behind it all: God wants what's best for His children.

WRAPPING UP

It would be easy to become self-condemning if we looked at our lives and focused only on the ways in which we've fallen short of being light to others. We must forget the negative past and move to the here and now. When we ask God to forgive our shortcomings. He forgives them and "throws them into the sea". That's why we must not relive a forgiven past. This limits our abilities to shine now and in the future for our Creator. What does it say about our God when we walk around heavy with guilt? Is this being a light or darkness to the world?

I want you to understand something. It would be impossible for us to be God's *lightful* representatives unless it was His plan and He'd made the way for it to be true. Here are two imperatives to remember:

- During day three of this week, we learned that Jesus makes it possible for us to become citizens of the Kingdom of light. He Himself makes us light by giving us His perfect relationship with God the Father.

- During day five of this week we learned how to keep our light shining brightly through daily following Jesus *the* Light.

Before we head into our day of rest, I want us to make sure we've grasped the transformational truths of this week into our beliefs.

- We need physical light for health. We have learned about the importance of the pro-hormone Vitamin D. We have learned how light governs the rhythms of the body, is an energy source and so much more.

- We heal as we leave stress and turn to God's rest, coming to Jesus.

- We can rest in His promise to bring us into His light. This is a gift for us to open.

- We can rest in His promise to make the changes we need to become His light to shine on others. Trust God to make the changes in us.

LIVING IN COMMUNITY

Talk with your study buddy about their plans to rest this week. Ask them how they keep their need to rest at the top of their mind and avoid stressing out about resting. Learn from them and share with them what you've found helps you.

BEING MISSIONAL

The day of rest reminds us of our need for God to be our everything, to be our light, to produce light in and through us. Be encouraging to someone in need. Be a light to those in a world of judgmentalism, negativity, and darkness. Watch their countenance change in the light of God's love shining through you. By His power, live the light He created you to be.

COMMITMENT

Today is a good day to transfer the Biblical Prescriptions for Life you've found especially useful to your master list on page vii. Today is also a great day to thank God for the ability in studying His Word with others, and for the ability to follow and trust Him.

DAY 7

Your Day of Rest

Use this space to record applicable notes about today's rest.

How did you invest it? _____

Where did you rest? _____

How did you join others in their rest? _____

How did you serve someone in an act of selfless love? _____

When you spent time in physical light, how did it feel? _____

What did you learn about God today? _____

What did you learn about yourself today? _____

Did the people you've been praying for come to your mind spontaneously? ____

Did you pray for them again? _____

Did you remember the physical importance of light? _____

What does light do for you physically? _____

Have you noticed areas of darkness in this world?_____

What are some ways you can bring light into darkness? _____

Sometimes the ministry of presence is all that is needed to bring light into an area. _____

In closing, we are just beginning to understand how light is so vital to our physiology. There is so much we do not know. Light is a universal truth. Make time for physical light. When out in the physical light, allow your brain to remind you of the perfect, life sustaining Light. Jesus is the Light of the world. Make time for this Light. Our goal is to learn to live in this Light one step at a time, one day at a time, encouraging each other along the journey.

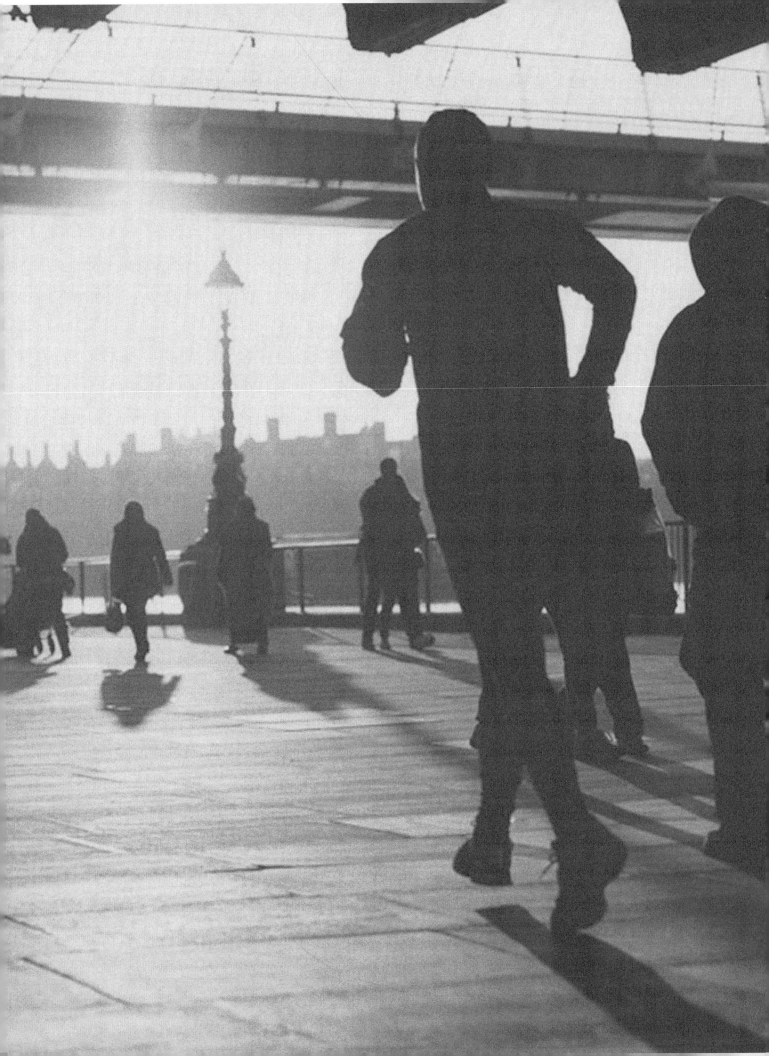

WEEK 4

Biblical Prescription for Life 3—God Created Us to Move

The Harris's have been married for 60 years. Both had experienced heart problems when they were in their seventies, but had done well. Last summer, they independently travelled to Alaska and enjoyed a trip of a lifetime.

But during the last few years, Mr. Harris had been suffering from arthritis and Mrs. Harris had been battling swelling (edema) of the legs. A few months ago, they were in the office where I explained that there was something missing in their lives that was more important than their daily medications. Since their body parts were more worn than they'd ever been before, they needed this missing ingredient now more than ever. The prescription they needed most was careful (but consistent) movement.

The human body ages at different rates, Mr. and Mrs. Harris, now in their eighties, had brains of sixty-year-olds. Mr. Harris's joints were more like those found in many ninety-year-olds as were the veins in Mrs. Harris's legs. I explained to them how important it was to not let their younger brains convince their "older" body parts to take on unreasonable activities. Notice the word "unreasonable." I wasn't saying that they needed to climb up on the roof to repair a few shingles, stand all day long, or even walk up stairs instead of taking an elevator. Such activities could put them at risk. Nor was I suggesting that they sit in a rocking chair all day. There was a vast middle ground waiting to bring help to their aging joints and veins.

I talked to them about *wisely* continuing to move all the parts. This was a key treatment to maintain their independence. As the nineties approached, they might have to modify their movement plan as balance could become a bit of a challenge.

To ease Mr. Harris's stiff and painful joints, I suggested that an activity like hourly stretching and walking with his cane would help keep his parts limber. "If you don't use it, you lose it," I said with a smile. This made sense to him. As a former engineer, he understood the importance of keeping moving things moving. Soon he was charting his stretching and steps, always being careful not to overdo. I explained how his movements were helping the ageing process by slowing oxidation, lengthening telomeres (the caps at the end of each strand of DNA that protect our chromosomes from the deterioration that hastens aging), and improving blood flow. Also by using the neuropathways involved in balance, his consistent movements were decreasing the risk of broken bones by improving balance and keeping the bones strong. No pill or medical treatment could quite accomplish this. I also explained the longer we sit and are inactive, the sooner our parts age—good advice for anyone of any age!

Mrs. Harris, not to be outdone, wished to join her husband on the road to better health. I explained that physical movement would keep her blood moving, lowering the risk of clots. Moving and stretching would also help the valves in her veins push the fluid out of her legs and reduce the swelling. This was one of the safest and cheapest treatments for venous insufficiency. She was immediately on board because she was definitely from the school of saving money.

Once I explained a few of the physiologic benefits of movement, they were committed. When I added that God designed us to move in order to keep our physiology at the optimum, they were even more committed, as they enjoyed a close relationship with their Creator.

Truth is a stubborn thing; it doesn't go away. Even though our bodies get older, more tired and stiff, and may suffer breakdowns occasionally, Biblical Prescriptions still apply. As we age, more care and creativity will be needed. In my case, I have noticed I need to rotate my movements and find myself spending more time in water, which lengthens my exercise before joint aches set in. The Harrises can't walk for prolonged lengths of time, but their regularity in short bouts of walking and stretching gives them great physiologic benefits.

I am glad to report that Mrs. Harris's edema has improved. Mr. Harris, while he still has some joint pain, reports that the moving and stretching regimen has reduced that pain to the point that he rarely has to take a mild pain medication.

Moving is a part of life, whether it's swimming, running, cycling, or walking. Being committed to daily following our original design will improve our lives at any age. We were not created to sit at a computer terminal or in a chair for prolonged periods of time. We were also designed for another daily exercise that brings about many physiologic benefits, a consistent and health-building walk with our Creator.

As we think about the importance of movement this week, I have another story to share that I hope will get us in the right frame of mind to improve our activity level this week.

Ted had a major heart attack 15 years ago. A non-smoker who did most things in moderation, his high-stress, relatively sedentary lifestyle put him at risk years before the crisis. Thankfully, God provided tremendous healing from the initial heart attack and Ted became committed to moving daily, thus changing every cell in his body. He also learned that a daily walk with God was the key to his health. He now enjoys walking while talking to and praising God. He understands that it's never too late to start walking, never too late to start improving, never too late to learn new truths and apply these truths. His biometrics (physical and behavioral characteristics) are better now than they were 20 years ago—well before his heart attack! By adding daily movement, his physical and spiritual life changed for the better.

As I discussed in our opening video, movement—even as simple as walking—improves every organ of our body by making our muscles, bone, blood vessels, and supporting structures work causing an improvement in circulation. Improved circulation means the organs are receiving a better supply of oxygen and nutrients with more efficient waste removal. Movement helps improve lung and muscle function and strengthens the heart. Exercising arm and leg muscles increases cellular respiration (the feeding, healing, and hygiene of our individual cells) by improving the arrival of nutrients and oxygen. By moving, we can decrease fat in the body, which helps prevent and treat diabetes and minimizes many other negative chemical reactions stemming from carrying excess weight.

Just look at this partial list of improvements brought about by consistent, daily movement:

- Improves brain function
- Stabilizes sleep patterns
- Improves digestion
- Enhances the circulatory system

- Increases joint mobility

- Develops muscle tone

- Enhances joint health

- Strengthens the bones

- Release endorphins which treat pain and diminish the stress chemistry

- Reduces the presence and effects of stress chemicals on the heart

The mainstay in the treatment of a weak heart is to give medications, which block the effects of stress chemicals on the heart. A daily movement program does exactly the same thing, plus all those other benefits!

I've just touched the surface of the many benefits of daily movement. In fact, science will continue to discover new healthy yields as technology improves. We're just now beginning to "measure" what God has promised from the beginning.

I can't say it enough: God designed our bodies to heal and be well as we follow His powerful and loving health plan! His ways create healing and wellness from head to foot. The best way to bring about that transformation is to commit to God's Biblical Prescriptions for Life. This week, we're going to adopt the healing power of movement into our lives.

VIDEO GUIDE 4

We're all Moving—Which Direction are You Going?

VIDEO (20 minutes)

Major Bible verses:

- Psalm 56:13

- Proverbs 3:5-6

Can you relate to the Harris's and Ted? With which you can most identify?

Age _____

Symptoms_____

Lifestyle_____

Relationships_____

What's the number one concern people have about making movement part of their lifestyle?

_____

What is the number one concern you have in making movement part of your life? _____

Does science support your concerns? _____

Remember: daily movement is responsible for *whole-body* health and the effective functioning of *every* system of the body. They're all interconnected, after all!

Let's review. Exposure to sunlight can improve vital bodily functions. What are they?

_____

_____

_____

Now, how about movement? Choose the benefit that meets your health concerns most and write it in the space provided:

Voluntary Muscle _____   _____

Heart Muscle _____   _____

Body leanness _____   _____

Stress Chemistry _____   _____

How much and which types of movement should we get each day?

Type of movement _____

Strenuousness of movement _____

Duration of movement _____

Review these realistic ways to add movement to your day. Then choose several to incorporate in your life starting today:

❑ Walk across the room or around the inside of your house/apartment each day for the next week

❑ Park farther away from your office door

❑ Using a pedometer, aim for 5,000 steps per day, then increase as you're able (15,000 steps is optimum)

❑ Every hour get up and move every body part.

❑ Walk outside (movement Rx + sunlight Rx) with your study buddy (relationship/community Rx's) and enjoy communing with God (worship Rx)

Think hard. Are there ways that a lack of movement might be negatively affecting your life right now?

_____

Movement—like every Biblical Prescription for Life—improves our entire body. Our chemistry, our metabolism, our strength, our energy, our cognition are all improved through daily movement.

Group Discussion (20 Minutes)

- Describe your mental mood after you've exercised?

- In what ways do you rest after you've put your body through a workout?

- When you don't exercise daily, how often do you feel sluggish or lethargic?

- How much time do you spend sedentary each day? Each week? Describe what you're doing.

- If you've ever started and then dropped a movement or exercise program, try to remember why you lost interest? What can you do to fix that problem and stay with the movement program?

- How can you balance your concerns about joint pain or difficulty moving with the science related to our body's need for movement each day?

- When was the last time you enjoyed moving or exercising? What were you doing and were you doing it with another person or group?

And now with your group, finish this sentence—"_I want to change _____"_

LIVING IN COMMUNITY

Congratulations! We're beginning our fourth week together, learning and adopting simple, scalable, sustainable Biblical Prescriptions for Life. Central to this study is the Biblical Prescription of relationships—our primary relationship with our loving Father and Creator and our secondary relationship with family, friends, and people who need family and friends.

Is there a fun or meaningful way you can share how someone in your study group has extended friendship to you? If so, please share. (Even if you don't share it in your group time today, take time to express your thankfulness to someone who has befriended you through _Biblical Prescriptions for Life._)

INDIVIDUAL REFLECTION

As we've listened to each other today, what is your top-level takeaway from this weeks' study so far? This is just for you. Write it here. _____

BEING MISSIONAL

Do you know someone who may believe that daily movement and exercise are unattainable goals? Write their name here _____ and contact them tomorrow. Encourage them to find some place to start. Be creative. Think about something appropriate for their current fitness level. It might be walking across their living room or it might be starting a "Couch to 5k" running plan with them.

God may use your initiative to help them overcome inertia (the tendency of an object at rest to stay at rest) in their body and their soul!

COMMITMENT

I want you to journal your movement each day. Keep track of movement and find ways to increase the time you spend moving. Also journal the amount of time you spend sitting. Be creative. Talk to your group. Encourage. I have given some specific daily challenges each day. As you keep this commitment, you will be blessed.

"This week, I am going to ADD and DO at least one of the following simple Biblical Prescriptions for Life:"

I commit to	My Biblical Prescription for Life	Day 1	2	3	4	5	6	7
	Read aloud 5x each day. Practice, memorize & recite:							
	Psalm 56:13 *"For You have delivered my soul from death, yes, my feet from falling, that I may walk before God in the light of life."*							
	Proverbs 3:5-6 *"Trust in the Lord with all your heart, and do not lean on your own understanding. In all your ways acknowledge him, and he will straight your paths."*							
	Movement 1							
	Movement 2							
	Movement 3							
	Movement 4							

If you missed a session or want to review one, go to biblicalprescriptionsforlife.com to stream Dr. Marcum's audio and video.

WEEK 4

It's Time to Put One Foot in Front of the Other

Healing involves treating the cause. Christ example should serve as our guide. He met needs, loved, and pointed those He served to a relationship with the Father. Healing is more than a quick fix. It's a journey that requires movement to arrive at a destination.

A few years ago I cared for a person who carried not only extra weight, but also extra burdens in life. He was searching for healing. He needed to understand that this was a journey and that he probably wouldn't be arriving at the destination by the end of the day. He also needed to understand how much he required the power and love that only comes through a relationship with Jesus. Such a one-step-at-a-time journey requires commitment as well.

As he walked with God, he was changed. The spiritual walk enabled the physical walk to have more meaning and value. In walking with Jesus, he understood how that relationship also changed his physiology.

As we think about movement this week, we must—as we have all along—move one step at a time, allowing God to change us from the inside out.

DAY 1

Choose to Get on the Path to Life

Movement is about direction. We decide to exert energy to move something *in a direction*. Whether or not we stay on course with the directional decision is determined by our resolve to:

- Keep moving.
- Keep making a host of smaller decisions consistent with the big decision.

Making choices inconsistent with your stated decision—or choosing not to choose—doesn't stop you from moving. It simply takes you off course.

Consider this example: If you want to go to the beach, you have to choose your destination and consider the logistics of how to make it happen. If you actually intend to *get* to the beach, you have to choose a route and then move forward along the route until you arrive at the beach! If you leave the course at the wrong exit, you'll most likely find yourself someplace *other* than the beach!

If you want to regain your health, you have to decide this is what you want—this is your destination. Remember our first week together? The Biblical Prescription for Life was facing Jesus' question that He directed at the man at the Pool of Bethesda. He looked him in the eye and asked, "Do you want to be healed?" This week, the focus is on the follow-up to that question—"Are you willing to take the steps necessary for healing to take place?"

It really is a choice. In His unsearchable wisdom and love for us, God gives you and me the gift of choice. Our ancestors, Adam and Eve, had the power to choose their course. Today, you and I also have the privilege and power to do the same.

Let's go to a place in the Bible where God brought His chosen people to a moment of decision. He was not asking them to choose blindly. Through His servant Moses, God makes the consequences of their choice—the path, the walk, the manner of living, and even the end results—very clear.

Mark the following words in the passages that follow:

- "walk" and "choose" with an arrow pointing to the right.

- "not" or equivalents with a red rectangle (red like a stop light) or a squiggly rectangle.

- any affirmative belief or action with a green rectangle (like a green light to proceed) or a straight rectangle.

You shall therefore love the Lord your God and keep his charge, his statutes, his rules, and his commandments always. And consider today (since I am not speaking to your children who have not known or seen it), consider the discipline of the Lord your God, his greatness, his mighty hand and his outstretched arm, his signs and his deeds that he did in Egypt to Pharaoh the king of Egypt and to all his land, and what he did to the army of Egypt, to their horses and to their chariots, how he made the water of the Red Sea flow over them as they pursued after you, and how the Lord has destroyed them to this day, and what he did to you in the wilderness, until you came to this place, and what he did to Dathan and Abiram the sons of Eliab, son of Reuben, how the earth opened its mouth and swallowed them up, with their households, their tents, and every living thing that followed them, in the midst of all Israel. For your eyes have seen all the great work of the Lord that he did.

You shall therefore keep the whole commandment that I command you today, that you may be strong, and go in and take possession of the land that you are going over to possess, and that you may live long in the land that the Lord swore to your fathers to give to them and to their offspring, a land flowing with milk and honey. For the land that you are entering to take possession of it is not like the land of Egypt, from which you have come, where you sowed your seed and irrigated it, like a garden of vegetables. But the land that you are going over to possess is a land of hills and valleys, which drinks water by the rain from heaven, a land that the Lord your God cares for. The eyes of the Lord your God are always upon it, from the beginning of the year to the end of the year.

And if you will indeed obey my commandments that I command you today, to love the Lord your God, and to serve him with all your heart and with all your soul, he will give the rain for your land in its season, the early rain and the later rain, that you may gather in your grain and your wine and your oil. And he will give grass in your fields for your livestock, and you shall eat and be full. Take care lest your heart be deceived, and you turn aside and serve other gods and worship them; then the anger of the Lord will be kindled against you, and he will shut up the heavens, so that there will be no rain, and the land will yield no fruit, and you will perish quickly off the good land that the Lord is giving you.

You shall therefore lay up these words of mine in your heart and in your soul, and you shall bind them as a sign on your hand, and they shall be as frontlets between your eyes. You shall teach them to your children, talking of them when you are sitting in your house, and when you are walking by the way, and when you lie down, and when you rise. You shall write them on the doorposts of your house and on your gates, that your days and the days of your children may be multiplied in the land that the Lord swore to your fathers to give them, as long as the heavens are above the earth. For if you will be careful to do all this commandment that I command you to do, loving the Lord your God, walking in all his ways, and holding fast to him, then the Lord will drive out all these nations before you, and you will dispossess nations greater and mightier than you. Every place on which the sole of your foot treads shall be yours. Your territory shall be from the wilderness to the Lebanon and from the River, the river Euphrates, to the western sea. No one shall be able to stand against you. The Lord your God will lay the fear of you and the dread of you on all the land that you shall tread, as he promised you.

See, I am setting before you today a blessing and a curse: the blessing, if you obey the commandments of the Lord your God, which I command you today, and the curse, if you do not obey the commandments of the Lord your God, but turn aside from the way that I am commanding you today, to go after other gods that you have not known. (Deuteronomy 11.1-28)

I call heaven and earth to witness against you today, that I have set before you life and death, blessing and curse. Therefore choose life, that you and your offspring may live, loving the Lord your God, obeying his voice and holding fast to him, for he is your life and length of days, that you may dwell in the land that the Lord swore to your fathers, to Abraham, to Isaac, and to Jacob, to give them. (Deuteronomy 30.19-20)

When God appointed Joshua to succeed Moses and take the Israelites into what would become the physical land of Israel's country, He had Joshua bring them to another point of decision. Keep marking like you did the passages from Deuteronomy.

Now therefore fear the Lord and serve him in sincerity and in faithfulness. Put away the gods that your fathers served beyond the River and in Egypt, and serve the Lord. And if it is evil in your eyes to serve the Lord, choose this day whom you will serve, whether the gods your fathers served in the region beyond the River, or the gods of the Amorites in whose land you dwell. But as for me and my house, we will serve the Lord. (Joshua 24.14-15)

God makes it abundantly clear that there is a monumental choice to make. What decision did God call His people the Israelites to make through Moses in Deuteronomy and again through Joshua in the book of Joshua? You'll see it quickly by looking at all of the arrows you marked. Write it here as simply as you can. _____

_____

Now, go back through the texts and look at all of the arrows you marked and record what God tells us are the outcomes of this choice:

If we choose to follow God	If we choose to walk any other way
Blessings	*Curses*

_____   _____
_____   _____
_____   _____
_____   _____
_____   _____
_____   _____

Does God want good things for us?

A list of outcomes like this can strike concern into our hearts. That's not all bad. I tell patients about the risks of cigarette smoking to give them a healthy concern of a very dangerous behavior. Choosing a life of selfishness and rebellion against our Loving Father is infinitely more dangerous than smoking cigarettes.

More motivating than concern of the negative outcomes, what does God tell us should drive our desire to follow Him?

_____

In your own words, explain the relationship between these momentous directional decisions and the hundreds of little decisions we make each day of our lives. Is following God a one-time decision or series of decisions—maybe even daily—or a combination? Please explain your answer.

_____
_____
_____
_____

WRAPPING IT UP

Is concern regarding negative outcomes a valid reason to make right choices? This is an important question. After all, abusers, dictators, tyrants, and terrorists use this in their attempt to control people. Two of the questions I ask when faced with concern are, "What's at stake?" and "Who or what is behind the threat?"

A bully can embarrass, intimidate, and even assault you physically. But there's always a larger authority we can appeal to as the threat rises. The intimidation they wield is often an influence we acquiesce to. But, even someone with the power and opportunity to kill me in a moment of lawlessness does not have ultimate authority of my ultimate destiny.

Jesus' disciples had good reason to have concerns. Following Jesus put them at odds with the religious rulers of Jerusalem--individuals who would persecute them and incite the Roman authorities against them. Knowing this, what did Jesus tell His disciples?

> So have no fear of them, for nothing is covered that will not be revealed, or hidden that will not be know. What I tell you in the dark, say in the light, and what you hear whispered, proclaim on the housetops. And do not fear those who kill the body but cannot kill the soul. Rather fear Him who can destroy both soul and body in hell. Are not two sparrows sold for a penny? And not one of them will fall to the ground apart from your Father. But even the hairs of your head are all numbered. Fear not, therefore; you are of more value than many sparrows. (Matthew 12.26-31)

God is no bully, tyrant or terrorist! He's our Heavenly Father and His love for us is perfect. He warns us of the terrible pain of moving away from Him in this life and the terrifying consequences in the next.

LIVING IN COMMUNITY

This might be a very good time to reach out to your study buddy and others in your group with the question: How has fear been used inappropriately in your life to harm you? What can you learn from that experience? How can you help each other identify *controlling fear*—fear that keeps you from moving toward God and others—from godly *fear* that keeps you from moving away from God and others?

BEING MISSIONAL

God is perfect. He knows when we need a warning and when we need an embrace. As you move toward God and others on this journey to healing and whole-life, life-long wellness, ask God for wisdom to know when and how to share His life-saving warnings. And remember, the reason why the gift of salvation Jesus offers to His followers is *good news* is because He saves us from the worst destiny imaginable to a new life with Him that will last forever.

COMMITMENT

Makes sure to review your commitments for week 4 and keep moving forward with your Biblical Prescriptions for Life from weeks 1 – 3. Remember, God will provide profound healing in your life through a relationship with Him and His people as you put simple, scalable, sustainable changes into everyday practice. You can do this! He will give you the power and joy to succeed!

Let's review. Do you understand where the answers to improving your health lie?

Are you drinking water and remembering the Living Water?

Make sure you move today. Are you writing down your movements? This will help you improve and realize the most efficient times and ways to move. Most find walking and stretching easy ways to move. Today, as you walk with God, appreciate nature and the grandeur of God's creation. Go outside if possible and really look around as you move. If you can't get outside, place a beautiful picture of God's creation someplace where you'll see it as you move by.

Choose this day, and every day, to walk with God.

DAY 2

Movement and the Walk of Life

Allow the physical movement of life to remind you of the importance of walking with God.

Every one of us is on a journey. In this physical life, it has a beginning marked by birth and an end marked by death. Each of us is moving from our personal physical beginning to our personal physical end. Unless Christ returns in our lifetime, each of all of us will experience death. That's a very sobering truth.

I see the reality of earthly death every day. I also see that each of us makes hundreds of small, seemingly insignificant choices each and every day that make profound impacts on that journey. Yes, there are the big decisions that we remember—momentous choices that dramatically direct our individual paths. Sometimes, our choices even affect the paths of others who are in a relationship with us. What few people realize is how our decisions are all interconnected. A "yes" to one option often creates a "no" to others. This means that every decision that we make changes our options in the future. Even fewer people realize that months and years of small choices add up to a way of life; that our decisions—both good and bad—move us through life. I want our movements through life to remind us of the importance of walking with God.

A big decision you may make during this seven-week study is to commit to a new way of thinking. That one decision will drive a new way of making thousands of subsequent choices.

Here's an example. I hope that one Biblical Prescription for Life that you've adopted is building healthy relationships. You might decide that living in meaningful relationships where you genuinely love one another through kindness, service, comfort, and compassion, is more valuable than living a life of selfishness. It's in community where we find healing.

That big decision will help you make seemingly smaller decisions such as:

- I will make the effort to initiate a personal visit with someone instead of getting distracted by social media.
- I will invest my resources into activities I can do with others instead of accumulating more stuff for myself.
- I will seek out time with my hurting friends to comfort them instead of leaving them alone so I don't have to get involved.
- I will become vulnerable and transparent about my own struggles as I help someone else find their way through a dark time instead of keeping up the appearance that I have it all together.

If you're consistent in your decision making and use it as the filter to move forward, those small decisions will become a way of life; a significant component of your personal (walk) journey. Your walk will become a blessing to many others who are in relationship with you. Your chosen Biblical Prescription for Life becomes a component of *their* journey as well. This is why studying *Biblical Prescriptions for Life* is so consistent with the way God intends for us to live. These prescriptions are personal, communal, and missional. God will transform your life, your community, and the world you live in as you embrace His perfect plan for you.

Journey. Movement. Walk. I want this physical motion to remind you to turn on brain pathways—your mental motions—constantly reminding you of your walk with God. Your daily decisions help determine your mental walk through life. Physical movement, mental movement, and walking with God are ways to lower the stress chemistry and serve as a treatment and perhaps prevent chronic disease.

Over the course of the previous three weeks, we've seen repeatedly how God uses the physical world to teach us great truths about the even "more real" spiritual world. The same is true with movement. Think about it. He could have made us stationary beings like a tree. Instead, he made us to move. And fundamentally, He made us to walk.

The simplest mode of an upright human being is walking. It's directional, taking you from point A to point B—unless you decide to walk in a circle! *Physical* walking is moving one step at a time. *Spiritual* walking is one thought, one decision, and one behavior at a time.

How we walk is supremely important to God. Will we walk in a loving relationship with Him? Here's some great news. God wants to teach us *how* to walk. It's such a big issue to Him that He brings the subject to the forefront nearly 200 times in the Old Testament and carries it prominently into the New Testament. When God returns to a topic this many times, it must be important. And if it's important to God, it must be important to His children.

Remember how God teaches us through comparisons and contrasts? He did it when He created light and darkness and when He created the earth below and the heavens above.

Today we're going to conclude with a brief look at what God has to say about the two ways to walk.

Mark these brief passages as you did yesterday:

- "walk" and "choose" with an arrow pointing to the right

- "not" or equivalents with the red rectangle (red like a stop light) or a squiggly rectangle.

- Any affirmation belief or action with a green rectangle (like a green light to proceed) or a straight rectangle

> Walk in a manner worthy of the LORD, to please Him in all respects, bearing fruit in every good work and increasing in the knowledge of God. (Colossians 1:10)

> So, as those who have been chosen of God, holy and beloved, put on a heart of compassion, kindness, humility, gentleness and patience; bearing with one another, and forgiving each other, whoever has a complaint against anyone; just as the Lord forgave you, so also should you. Beyond all these things put on love, which is the perfect bond of unity. Let the peace of Christ rule in your hearts, to which indeed you were called in one body; and be thankful. Let the word of Christ richly dwell within you, with all wisdom teaching and admonishing one another with psalms and hymns and spiritual songs, singing with thankfulness in your hearts to God. Whatever you do in word or deed, do all in the name of the Lord Jesus, giving thanks through Him to God the Father. (Colossians 3:12-17)

For we are His workmanship, created in Christ Jesus for good works, which God prepared beforehand, that we should walk in them. (Ephesians 2:10)

Walk in a manner worthy of the calling with which you have been called. (Ephesians 4:1)

Let no unwholesome word proceed from your mouth, but only such a word as is good for edification according to the need of the moment, so that it will give grace to those who hear. Do not grieve the Holy Spirit of God, by whom you were sealed for the day of redemption. Let all bitterness and wrath and anger and clamor and slander be put away from you, along with all malice. Be kind to one another, tenderhearted, forgiving each other, just as God in Christ also has forgiven you. (Ephesians 4:29-32)

I appeal to you therefore, brothers, by the mercies of God, to present your bodies as a living sacrifice, holy and acceptable to God, which is your spiritual worship. Do not be conformed to this world, but be transformed by the renewal of your mind, that by testing you may discern what is the will of God, what is good and acceptable and perfect. (Romans 12:1-2)

Who is the man who fears the LORD? Him will He instruct in the way that he should choose. (Psalm 25:12)

Your word is a lamp to my feet and a light to my path. (Psalm 119:105)

Trust in the LORD with all your heart, and do not lean on your own understanding, in all your ways acknowledge Him and He will make straight your paths. (Proverbs 3:5-6)

Then they will call upon Me, but I will not answer; they will seek Me diligently but will not find Me. Because they hated knowledge and did not choose the fear of the LORD, would have none of My counsel and despised all My reproof. (Proverbs 1:28-30)

And by this we know that we have come to know Him, if we keep His commandments. Whoever says, 'I know Him' but does not keep His commandments is a liar, and the truth is not in him, but whoever keeps His word, in him truly the love of God is perfected. By this we may know that we are in Him: whoever says he abides in Him ought to walk in the same way in which He walked. (1 John 2:3-6)

If My people who are called by My name humble themselves, and pray and seek My face and turn from their wicked ways, then I will hear from heaven and will forgive their sin and heal their land. (2 Chronicles 7:14)

I will meditate on Your precepts and fix my eyes on Your ways. (Psalm 119:15)

There are two ways to walk. List what you learn about walking...

...God's way:	...or any other way
_____	_____
_____	_____
_____	_____
_____	_____

_____   _____

_____   _____

_____   _____

_____   _____

Summarize in your own words what God is trying to tell us about how we walk.

_____

Who makes the choice about the way we live? _____

Your walk is your manner of life. Tomorrow, we're going to dig deep into what God wants us to know about spiritual walking. He loves us and wants us to experience joy, healing, and wholeness. That's why He has written His instructions to us and saved them in the Bible so we—and everyone else—can know Him and His ways.

WRAPPING IT UP

Have you thought about the path you're on? None of us are staying in one place. Even someone who is severely restricted in movement to the point of being confined to their bed makes choices about what they will believe, how they will choose, and what they will do. Imagine the person who believes God has forgotten them and descends into the darkness of self-pity compared to the person who takes God at His promises—that He loves them and will never forsake them—and chooses to be a force of encouragement in every human interaction they enjoy.

Looking back, you can already recall milestones in your life that set or altered your journey. You may see with regret how there were some areas in your life where "choosing not to choose" kept you on a course that months and years later brought you to a place that wasn't healthy.

The great news is that God's mercies are new every day! Today, you can take steps on the path toward healing and life-long, whole life wellness.

LIVING IN COMMUNITY

Biblical Prescriptions for Life is a program centered on our loving God who gives us clear, perfect direction for living life—now and eternally—to the fullest.

It's my prayer for you that you are developing some of the best, most constructive relationships of your life through embarking on this journey together with your small group. I encourage you to be transparent and vulnerable with your Study Buddy or someone else in your group. Call them when you can both talk and share something you've been doing that has put you on a course you now want to change. It can be something big. Or, it can be a pattern of small things. But take the risk and let your Study Buddy into your life at that deeper level. You may be surprised to find you're not alone.

BEING MISSIONAL

One of God's most praise-worthy characteristics is His mercy. He loves us. He forgives us. He gives us new ways to think and the power to change our beliefs, choices, and actions. I'm eternally grateful!

As you continue to learn truths from God and start to discern between healthy and unhealthy beliefs and choices, it's crucial that you exercise mercy in the way that you share what you're learning. Most people haven't had their beliefs challenged as yours have been challenged during the past three weeks. Be prayerful, gentle, and wise in what and when you share. Make sure God is telling you to approach someone about an expressed belief or a demonstrated behavior before you do it. Then be as merciful and loving toward them as you would want someone to be toward you. Being judgmental is more dangerous than smoking a pack of cigarettes or drinking too many sugary drinks.

COMMITMENT

For many people, adopting a movement way of life is a challenge. Remember to scale the Biblical Prescriptions for Life you choose this week. Don't go from couch to marathon in one leap. You'll hurt yourself, discourage yourself, and potentially give up altogether. Your initial commitment might be to just get up from the chair and move every hour or it might be to stretch out and deep breathe every hour. For some it might be walking for forty-five minutes a day. Start somewhere you can find success and build from there.

When in doubt, talk it out. Share your choices with your Study Buddy. Then make time to encourage him or her in their commitments.

Pause now and transfer your Biblical Prescriptions for Life from week three to page vii, with your running list of sustainable changes. Look at what God is doing in and through you already! Thank Him for His kindness and care for you. You are on your way to healing.

Today as you go on your walk/movement, I want you to specifically focus on talking to God. Yesterday you focused on nature and the grandeur of God. Today, just talk. As you focus on the physical and link it to the spiritual, there will be synergistic benefits to your physiology. Our goal is to have every movement remind us of our relationship with God. This might be on a subconscious level, but we want the movements of our mind focused on our Creator. Write your movements and how you are feeling in your journal. Look back on previous days to determine what is working best for you.

DAY 3

Two Ways to Walk

Today, let's focus on trusting God's way for us to walk. Let's learn to allow Him to define the movements of our life.

Last week, we discovered how our thoughts, decisions, and actions are built on underlying beliefs whether those beliefs are accurate or not, true or false, light or darkness, or righteous or sinful. They may be healthy, healing, and life giving, or selfish, destructive, and deadly.

Yesterday we became aware that these thoughts, decisions, and actions become our manner of living. They become our way of life. The Bible refers to this as our "walk."

We saw how our loving Father did not create robots without a will. Rather, He blessed us with the awesome responsibility to choose how we walk. And true to His perfect wisdom and total love for us, He gives us a preview of the very different journeys that follow our choices as well as providing an encouragement—or warning as the case may be—of the ultimate destination for each. Hundreds and thousands of little, seemingly insignificant, and unrelated choices become our lifestyle. We'll all look back one day and see how we paved the path for our destiny.

Have you been making good choices? Are you on a safe path? Why not let God take control of the movements of your life. Who knows you better than your Creator? Who knows the best plan for you?

If you recognize that your path is dangerous—be thankful! Thankful that your loving Father has alerted you and given you a path to safety.

As long as it is still "today," God gives you and me the choice afresh. Remember Joshua's call to choose?

"Choose for yourself today whom you will serve". (Joshua 24:15) Along with that choice comes a promise. God will provide grace as we stumble along the way,

> The steadfast love of the LORD never ceases; His mercies never come to an end; they are new every morning; great is Your faithfulness. (Lamentations 3:22-23)
>
> Delight yourself in the LORD, and He will give you the desires of your heart. Commit your way to the LORD; trust in Him, and He will act. He will bring forth your righteousness as the light, and your justice as the noonday. (Psalm 37:4-6)

I have a close friend who describes God's balance of warnings and encouragements this way. He says that on the journey of life, God's warnings are like the center stripe and the white line painted on the road and guardrails on each side. His promises to bless us are like the well-lit horizon laid out clearly before us. When life is foggy and the weather is inclement, the center stripe and white line keep us in our lane while the guardrails prevent us from going headlong into the ditch. You can't drive fast when you have low-to-no visibility. You tend to weave ever so slightly as the road unfolds ten or twenty meters at a time.

On sunny days and clear nights, the unobstructed view of the horizon allows us to move forward at top speed with anticipation and excitement. We can travel with confidence and purpose. Our movements are fluid and confident.

God wants us to move forward with Him. He lovingly provides warnings to keep us on the road when things aren't clear and our will to choose between selfishness and love is at war within us. As we allow Him to define our movements, trust will grow.

Let's stop right now and thank God for making these provisions for us so we can walk decisively with Him..

With more than 200 examples and instructions regarding the way to walk revealed in the pages of the Bible, we can't possibly go through all of them here. Yet, it's vitally important that we look at some highlights. After all, the power of *Biblical Prescriptions for Life* is not in what I say. It's not even in what your study buddy or small group say. The only power for real change resides within the Spirit of God, defining the movements in your life as you allow the truths of the Bible to change what you believe. Only the Spirit will motivate you toward those life-giving choices, which change you physically as you trust God to lead you one-step at a time.

Let's learn directly from our loving Father, the Great Physician, about the blessings He freely gives to those who walk in His ways.

> And if you will walk in My ways, keeping My statutes and My commandments, as your father David walked, then I will lengthen your days. (1 Kings 3:14)
>
> Therefore, you shall keep the commandments of the Lord your God, to walk in His ways and to fear Him. (Deuteronomy 8:6)
>
> He has told you, O man, what is good; and what does the LORD require of you but to do justice, and to love kindness, and to walk humbly with your God? (Micah 6:8)
>
> Blessed is the man who walks not in the counsel of the wicked, nor stands in the way of sinners, nor sits in the seat of scoffers; but his delight is in the law of the LORD, and on His law he meditates day and night. He is like a tree planted by streams of water that yields its fruit in its season, and its leaf does not wither. In all that he does he prospers. (Psalm 1:1-3)

Yesterday we learned there are benefits—blessings or "joyful conditions"—of following God and His way of living; His perfect plan for us. This is walking with God.

There are two ways to walk. List what you learn about walking...

...God's way:	**...or any other way**
_____	_____
_____	_____
_____	_____
_____	_____
_____	_____
_____	_____

_____   _____

_____   _____

Summarize in your own words how God is defining walking with Him for you.

_____

Who makes the choice about the way we live?   _____

Please take time right now to capture in words what God is showing you through today's study. Take this moment to contemplate your life and His calling for you to joyfully choose to follow Him.

WRAPPING IT UP

Remember what God taught us about light from our _Biblical Prescription for Life_ study from last week? It's beautiful how many times God puts the idea of movement—walking, living, and being—in the context of light. Light represents truth, the purity of God and His presence; of being fully known and living in complete honesty, as we love God and one another; staying out of the darkness of lies, broken beliefs, and selfishness.

He designed us to live a lifestyle of light, in His presence, following His perfect plan for us, serving others in community and on a mission to introduce others to the Light. God is calling us to walk in the light today, to travel on the journey of life with Him and to move toward Him and others in love.

LIVING IN COMMUNITY

I appreciate excellent, life-enriching poetry. Whether it's written, spoken, or put to music, poetry helps us think in fresh ways about things we may overlook.

God is the Ultimate Physician. He is also the Ultimate Poet. Consider that He speaks to us in physical terms to teach us concerning profound, eternally important, supremely significant spiritual truths. He has made our bodies to walk. He created light and darkness for us to experience contrast. And He makes exposure to the sun physiologically necessary and beneficial.

Invite your Study Buddy—and maybe a few others from your _Biblical Prescriptions for Life_ study group—out for a walk this week. Schedule it today so you can all slip it into your busy schedules. Then enjoy moving together toward God and in His joyful presence on the journey of life.

BEING MISSIONAL

Here's a way you can reach someone who's not yet walking with God: you can invite him or her to walk with you! Getting your neighbor out for a daily walk around the block will build a relationship platform from which you can share what you're learning about this sublime journey toward life-long wellness.

COMMITMENT

You have two places to find your Biblical Prescriptions for Life. 1. The simple actions you choose this week after watching the video on movement with your group. 2. The master list you've been updating as you've collected the prescriptions that allow you to move forward in your life.

Hopefully, your movement journal is becoming a habit. Today, however, I want you to commit to something specific during your physical walk/movement. I want you to focus on praising God as you physically move. Concentrate on His many blessings and thank Him for all that He has done and is doing for you.

Make sure you're also keeping up the new habits of renewing your mind through Bible memory and recitation. Your life is being transformed! Enjoy the journey.

DAY 4

"Works" and "Fruit"—the Evidence of Movement

We may not understand where our walk is taking us until we get there.

We've set the stage for the two competing lifestyles existing in the cosmos—God's way and any other way. God's way is described as "being in the light" and being in His presence; growing, healing, experiencing life to the fullest. Any other way will bring hardship in this life. Even materially wealthy people who don't follow God experience relational poverty and the absence of peace.

When we're moving with God, we may not understand where our path is going until we get there. The reason is simple. As sinful human beings, we can't fully understand God. However, the more we move with Him and see how He leads, the more our faith will grow. God will give us evidence that He is with us, guiding us along the journey. We may not understand God, but we can comprehend His presence in our lives.

In this God-directed "walk of life," choices are made that generate the movements of life, hundreds and thousands of seemingly small and insignificant choices that serve to keep us on course. The same can be said about walking on any other path that begs the questions, "How do we know when we're on the right path?"

Movement begins in our mind where our beliefs, will, and emotions live. As we will study in week six, the Biblical Prescription for Life also deals with our mind, what we think about and desire. We will get the right start by letting God renew our minds that will, in turn, determine our beliefs, will, and emotions.

Let's ask God to search our hearts as we dig into today's study.

> Create in me a clean heart, O God, and renew a right spirit within me. (Psalm 51:10)
>
> Search me, O God, and know my heart! Try me and know my thoughts! And see if there be any grievous way in me, and lead me in the way everlasting! (Psalm 139:23-24)
>
> Do not be anxious about anything, but in everything by prayer and supplication with thanksgiving let your requests be made known to God. And the peace of God, which surpasses understanding, will guard your hearts and your minds in Christ Jesus. (Philippians 4:6-7)
>
> For though we walk in the flesh (meaning, live life in a physical body in this occurrence), we are not waging war according to the flesh. For the weapons of our warfare are not of the flesh but have divine power to destroy strongholds. We destroy arguments and every lofty opinion raised against the knowledge of God, and take every thought captive to obey Christ. (2 Corinthians 10:3-5:)

I'm so astounded that the Creator of the universe wants to develop a relationship with me *and* He wants to lead me on the path to ultimate joy, satisfaction, meaning, purpose, and yes, *wellness*. He wants to lead us. He wants to speak to us!

Even though God desires to lead us, He still lets us choose whether we want to be led. And, if you're like me, there have been times in your life when you've made selfish decisions that you were able to justify. That's why God warned us to be careful about justifying, rationalizing, and tricking ourselves into minimizing our selfishness. Oh, the wisdom of God!

God's prophet Jeremiah wrote about this self-trickery in Jeremiah 17:9: "The heart is deceitful above all things, and desperately sick; who can understand it?" But, don't be discouraged by the past. Be encouraged! God wants to safeguard us from self-deceit as we make present and future decisions.

> Trust in the LORD with all your heart, and do not lean on your own understanding. In all your ways acknowledge Him and He will make straight your paths. Do not be wise in your own eyes; fear the LORD, and turn away from evil. It will be healing to your flesh and refreshment to your bones. (Proverbs 3:5-8)

How do we know if we're walking with God in His light as opposed to walking any other way?

Just as God has made knowing the right starting place clear, we can also know when we're on the right path. He's provided a way for our in-the-light lifestyle to become evident to us as well as the people with whom we enjoy a relationship.

When walking away from God becomes evident:

Like a blood test that reveals warning signs, God gives us clear indications to know which way we're headed on our journey—and what decisions are directing us.

> But I say, walk by the Spirit and you will not gratify the desires of the flesh [our sinful nature since Adam]. For the desires of the flesh are against the Spirit, and the desires of the Spirit are against the flesh, for these are opposed to each other, to keep you from doing the things you want to do [this is the war inside us all between selfishness and godliness]. But if you are led by the Spirit, you are not under the law. Now the works of the flesh are evident: sexual immorality, impurity, sensuality, idolatry, sorcery, enmity, strife, jealousy, fits of anger, rivalries, dissensions, division, envy, drunkenness, orgies, and things like these. I warn you, as I have warned you before, that those who do such things will not inherit the kingdom of God. (Galatians 5:16-21; my comments added)

God's movement in us and through us creates growth:

God gives a very clear way to know when we're moving away from Him (walking in darkness) or walking toward Him (walking in His light). As we walk in Him, He creates movement in and through us. Like life-carrying sap flowing from the branches of a grape plant through the vine, God Himself produces spiritual fruit—the "Fruit of the Spirit"—in and through us. .

> But the fruit of the Spirit is love, joy, peace, patience, kindness, goodness, faithfulness, gentleness, self-control; against such things there is no law. And those who belong to Christ Jesus have crucified the flesh with its passions and desires. If we live by the Spirit, let us also keep in step with the Spirit. (Galatians 5:22-25)

> And I am sure of this, that He who began a good work in you will bring it to completion at the day of Jesus Christ. (Philippians 1:6)

> For it is God who works in you, both to will and to work for His good pleasure. (Philippians 2:13)

Let's make two lists—one of the deeds of the flesh (which come out of us when we walk any way other than God's way), and the fruit of Spirit (which grow out of us when we walk God's way).

Works of the Flesh	Fruit of the Spirit
_____	_____
_____	_____
_____	_____
_____	_____
_____	_____
_____	_____

Which way do you think would bring the most profound blessedness (literally, "joyful condition") to you and to the ones in your life? _____

Which evidences do you see most in your life today? _____

What would your spouse, best friend or co-workers say about you? _____

Why do you think that is happening? _____

Do you feel that you are moving away from God or toward Him? _____

Why do you say that? _____

Let's pause to talk to God right now. Ask Him to search your heart and bring to awareness any belief, desire, or feeling that's selfish, unhealthy, or contrary to His character and the truth He has taught you.

> *Father, You love me more than I'll ever realize. You give me your good instructions to keep me safe and on the path to life. Thank You for showing me where I'm not moving toward You. I want to stop _____ (use specific language here—don't be vague) and start trusting and obeying You with my beliefs, thoughts, desires, emotions, and actions. Thank You for forgiving me for my selfishness and sin. Thank You for giving me power over selfishness and sin so that I may follow you. Thank You that You don't condemn me. Rather, You love me back to wholeness. Amen.*

WRAPPING IT UP

We're always moving. *Always.* And either we're moving away from God or toward Him. That movement which begins in our thoughts, will, and emotions eventually shows up in the choices we make, the words we say, and the things we do.

When I feel a lack of the Fruit of the Spirit or when my family notices that lack in me, it's time for me to stop and reconnect with my perfect Father. He wants only the absolute best for me. He wants me back and will never turn me away. Remember each day is a new day. We cannot live in the past. We live one day at a time. We walk one decision at a time. We move one step at a time.

LIVING IN COMMUNITY

This is a good time to text your study buddy about the wonderful things God has shown us today. Think purposefully and try to identify one or more evidences of the God's Fruit in their life that you've experienced by knowing them. Then encourage them by telling them about it. Spiritual fruit is significant because it's proof positive that God is living in and flowing through them. He is creating the most important movement in their life!

BEING MISSIONAL

Few things are as attractive in a friend as the Fruit of the Spirit. Why are you patient when others are demanding? Why do you have joy even when things aren't going perfectly for you? Why do you stick with someone through hard times? Why do you love instead of "looking out for number One"?

Whether we realize it or not, someone is always watching us. When the time is right, they'll say something to you and ask you to tell them about what makes you different. With the Apostle Peter, be ready to share God's love— "But in your hearts honor Christ the Lord as holy, always being prepared to make a defense to anyone who asks you for a reason for the hope that is in you; yet do it with gentleness and respect". (1 Peter 3.15)

COMMITMENT

Review your running list of Biblical Prescriptions for Life with this week's additions. Keep it simple and keep at it. Studies show that after 30 to 45 days of practice, choices (good or bad) become habits. Are your journal entries helping you stay on track?

Today as you walk, move, stretch, or swim, I want you to give thanks as you move. Make this your focus. After your movement, ask yourself: How did talking to God and praising Him make me feel? Do I notice anything different?"

Remember, as we walk with God, we may not understand where the walk is going, but there will be evidence that God is leading.

DAY 5

Daily, ask God to walk with us

Yesterday, during our time together, we learned how we could evaluate our walk. We should honestly ask whether we act:

- Selfishly—what the Bible calls "in the flesh" where we prioritize our own self-centered, self-promoting, self-protecting, self-providing interests at the expense of following God or loving others

- Godwardly—what the Bible calls "in the Spirit" where we walk in the power of God's Spirit with our desires fixed on loving Him and loving others

We learned that God has given us a diagnostic tool so we can detect when we've begun to move away from His pathway toward anything else. Like taking your blood pressure, Galatians 5:19-25 offers two contrasting lists that outline the symptoms of moving toward or away from God. Try your best to summarize them here:

Symptoms that demonstrate I'm moving away from God; becoming selfish:

_____

_____

Symptoms that demonstrate I'm moving toward God; becoming loving:

_____

_____

Be honest. What did you detect about your life? Do you look normal on the outside, but inside you're struggling between being self-ward and being Godward? Don't worry. That's very normal. It's actually very encouraging. Even the apostle Paul identified that struggle in his own life.

> I find then a law, that evil is present with me, the one who wills to do good. For I delight in the law of God according to the inward man. But I see another law in my members, warring against the law of my mind, and bringing me into captivity to the law of sin, which is in my members. O wretched man that I am! Who will deliver me from this body of death? I thank God—through Jesus Christ our Lord! So then, with the mind I myself serve the law of God, but with the flesh the law of sin. (Romans 7:21-15)

A fever can be evidence that your body is fighting an infection. Fever, an elevated white blood cell count, and redness and swelling are all physical responses indicating that your immune system is hard at work fighting disease. If you didn't experience the discomfort of these responses, you'd not realize your body was working to fight the offending agent. In many cases, symptoms—as uncomfortable as they may be—can be a very good thing. I'd rather know I was sick so I could realize my true state of health and do something about it.

As we've seen throughout *Biblical Prescriptions for Life*, physical conditions can mirror spiritual realities.

As Paul discovered, the struggle between selfishness and love is evidence that we're alive. If God were not working in your life, there'd be no struggle. Thanks to Adam, selfishness comes naturally, and unless God demonstrated a better way that was actually *more* fulfilling, you'd never know the difference. You'd never want to live any other way. Like our sin-sick DNA, our desires default to selfishness *unless* we seek our loving Father and the Ultimate Physician through prayer and daily Bible study. We must continually ask God to keep us on the right path, accomplishing *His* will, not ours.

Remember, we get pointed in the right direction through coming into the light and letting God renew our minds. However, we must take some action. There are choices needing to be made each and every day.

How do we know when to ask God to keep us on track? How do we get back on track? How do we stop moving away from God, turn and start moving toward Him? Think back through what we've learned so far.

- In week 1 we heard Jesus ask, "Do you really want to be made well?" In response, we ask ourselves, "Do I acknowledge that God is the Ultimate Physician, or am I too busy to care? Do I want to come and worship God? Do I agree that Jesus is the only hope that I have of spiritual healing? Will I accept His healing rest?"

- In week 2 we learned that Jesus would give us the living water to flow through us. He alone can create life in our souls and change our direction.

- In week 3 we learned that living in the light is where God is. When we confess our selfishness to God and to those we've hurt, He forgives us and cleanses us from our guilt. He restores us to a right relationship with Him. He brings us back into the light.

Now in week four, we're learning that we are constantly in movement. If you find yourself moving—in thoughts, desires, or actions—away from a loving God and others, then put the Biblical Prescriptions for Life from weeks 1-3 in practice and move back toward Him. Renew your mind. Seek Him first. Trust, listen, and then follow Him. This needs to be done daily. Ask God daily to walk with you.

You and I are truly moving— moving toward God. Read the following passages and mark:

- Anything we are supposed to stop, let go of, or avoid with an oval and an arrow pointed down or an octagon like stop sign.
- Any action word such as "walk", "run", return", "seek" "draw near" with an arrow pointed to the right.

When heaven is shut up and there is no rain because they have sinned against you, if they pray toward this place and acknowledge Your name and turn from their sin, when You afflict them, then hear in heaven and forgive the sin of Your servants, Your people Israel, when You teach them the good way in which they should walk, and grant rain upon Your land, which You have given to you Your people as an inheritance. (2 Chronicles 6:26-27)

I have blotted out your transgressions like a cloud and your sins like a mist; return to Me, for I have redeemed you. (Isaiah 44:22)

Seek the LORD while He may be found; call upon Him while He is near; let the wicked forsake his way, and the unrighteous man his thoughts; let him return to the LORD, that He may have compassion on him, and to our God, for He will abundantly pardon. For My thoughts are not your thoughts, neither are your ways My ways, declares the LORD. For as the heavens are higher that the earth, so are My ways higher than your ways and My thoughts than your thoughts. (Isaiah 55:6-9)

Therefore say to them, thus declares the LORD of hosts: Return to Me, says the LORD of hosts, and I will return to you, says the LORD of hosts. (Zechariah 1:3)

"Yet even now," declares the LORD, "return to Me with all your heart, with fasting, with weeping, and with mourning; and rend your hearts and not your garments." Return to the LORD your God, for He is gracious and merciful, slow to anger, and abounding in steadfast love. (Joel 2:12-13)

Brothers, I do not consider that I have made it (Paul is speaking of his right standing with God) my own. But one thing I do" forgetting what lies behind and straining forward to what lies ahead, I press on toward the goal for the prize of the upward call of God in Christ Jesus. Let those of us who are mature think this way, and if in anything you think otherwise, God will reveal that also to you. Only let us hold true to what we have obtained. Brothers, join in imitating me, and keep your eyes on those who walk according to the example you have in us. (Philippians 3:13-17)

Therefore, since we are surrounded by so great a cloud of witnesses, let us also lay aside every weight, and sin which clings so closely, and let us run with endurance the race that is set before us, looking to Jesus, the founder and perfecter of our faith, who for the joy that was set before Him endured the cross, despising the shame, and is seated at the right hand of the throne of God. (Hebrews 12:1-2)

For bodily discipline is only of little profit, but godliness is profitable for all things, since it holds promise for the present life and also for the life to come. (1 Timothy 4:8)

If then you have been raised with Christ, seek the things that are above, where Christ is, seated at the right hand of God. Set your minds on things that are above, not on things that are on earth. (Colossians 3:1-4)

But He gives more grace. Therefore it says, 'God opposes the proud, but gives grace to the humble.' Submit yourselves therefore to God. Resist the devil and he will flee from you. Draw near to God, and He will draw near to you. (James 4:6-8)

But as for you, O man of God, flee these things (craving wealth and possessions). Pursue righteousness, godliness, faith, love, steadfastness, and gentleness. Fight the good fight of the faith. Take hold of the eternal life to which you were called and about which you made the good confession in the presence of many witnesses. (1 Timothy 6:11-12; my explanation added)

Now, fill in these three lists based on the above texts.

...What we're moving away from	...and what we're moving toward	...and He will

Examine your lists closely and answer these questions:

Are we ever instructed to leave or drop anything that's actually good for us?

_____

We're even instructed to leave our self-righteousness behind (Philippians 3). Why might God want us to do this?

_____

What on the list of things we're called toward is most appealing to you? Why?

_____

_____

Now, with complete honesty, do you believe that God's ways are the best for you? Why?

_____

_____

God loves us more than we can understand or imagine. Think of how much you love your parents, your spouse, or your children. They can't possibly know the depth of love you have for them. Then think about the infinitely good, infinitely loving, infinitely powerful Creator of the universe and how His love for us must be infinitely greater than our finite minds could contain.

Contemplate this text prayerfully:

> If you then, being evil, know how to give good gifts to your children, how much more will your heavenly Father give the Holy Spirit to those who ask Him? (Luke 11:13)

WRAPPING IT UP

I'm so thankful to God that, not only does He love me perfectly, but He also loves me enough to give me clear, loving instruction on how to live symptom free! He's the perfect Father, the Ultimate Physician. And He wants you and me to learn to live by His Biblical Prescriptions for Life.

Let's stop and thank Him for providing a way to return to Him and get back on the path to healing and whole-life, lifelong wellness.

LIVING IN COMMUNITY

If through a selfish act—more than just a thought or desire—you have hurt someone, I encourage you to seek a God to help you determine if you need to make things right with that person. You may need to find a way to make restitution. This is tough. But, God is stronger than tough. He promises freedom for those who turn from selfishness and move toward Him.

BEING MISSIONAL

God forgives! What could be better news than the fact that God forgives people who turn to Him. This "good news" is known as the Gospel. It's God's way of rescuing mankind from pursuing their own selfish interests that can lead them to eternal harm.

Is there someone you know that needs to know God? Do you know someone who could benefit from a forgiving spirit and an invitation to enjoy a healthy, healing relationship? Maybe it's someone you've been praying for and reaching out to through weeks one, two and three.

COMMITMENT

How are you doing with your Biblical Prescriptions for Life? Are you meditating on the Bible verses? Are you able to recite a few from memory? How is God bringing them to mind during the day?

This week we've been focusing on the physical act of moving or exercise. Have you been adding a few exercises to your daily routine? I hope by journaling and focusing on movement, this is becoming a habit in your routine. Have you deliberately moved each day this week? Are you figuring out ways to incorporate daily movement? For some this might be a habit at which we really have to work. Just know there will be physical and spiritual benefits.

Today, your assignment is to walk while thinking of ways you can serve others. If you really want to multi-task, drink a glass of water and then walk in the sunshine with one of your friends.

Make sure to keep moving forward with your work. Don't become overwhelmed. Take it one step at a time. Encourage your classmates. It takes weeks to form new habits. While you're being faithful to your practice of each prescription, you are re-wiring your neural pathways and bringing true healing from the inside out. Your physiology and chemistry is changing. God is adjusting more than one chemical pathway. He's accomplishing much more than treating a symptom. He's changing a life. *Your* life. This is exciting!

DAY 6

Walking with God is Joyous, Fulfilling, and Free

Sometimes, I find it's very helpful to share with others examples of success—without disclosing personally identifiable information. This may encourage patients and others on their journey to wellness, especially when the road ahead seems difficult or when they're experiencing a slow recovery or face a setback. God made us for relationships. One of those types of relationships includes learning from people who've gone before and how others have walked with God.

The nation of Israel's second king was a man named David. You may have heard about him. His story begins when, as a small shepherd boy, he defeats the God-cursing giant Goliath using a simple sling and a smooth, round stone.

You can read his story in the books of 1 Samuel, 2 Samuel, 1 Kings, and 1 Chronicles. You'll also find David's conversations with and about God—and hear his heart speak in raw truth—in the book of Psalm. David himself wrote most of the Psalms.

God had chosen David to be King because he was, as God described him, "a man after my own heart," (Acts 13.22). He was far from perfect and some of his acts of disobedience were quite spectacular. His errors in judgment and moral improprieties cost David, his family, and his people dearly. But what is most telling about David is that he loved God. And when he found himself moving away from Him, he repented (literally, "changed his mind" and turned direction) and followed God again.

What set David apart was the movement of his heart toward his heavenly Father. He sought God. This goes right to the heart of the matter—literally and figuratively. God made us for a relationship with Himself and with each other. He wants to satisfy us. But, He wants us to want Him more than anything or anyone else. That sounds megalomaniacal unless you take God at His word. Our Father represents perfect love, perfect goodness, and perfect power. No human can be those things. When we find God, we've discovered more than we could ever hope or imagine. Walking with Him will bring happiness, fulfillment, and is a free gift. David wrote: "You make known to me the path of life; in Your presence there is fullness of joy; at Your right hand are pleasures forevermore" (Psalm 16.11). No human can offer that level of satisfaction and joy.

That's why I hope each one of us can say, "I want to know God and be with Him more than anything else. Being with God is my life's ambition."

Let's spend our time today being encouraged by other hearts moving toward God.

Mark the following passages this way:

- The word "seek" with an arrow pointed to the right

- Draw a triangle on "God" and pronouns for Him

- Draw a green rectangle around the reasons and blessings listed for seeking God

> O God, you are my God; earnestly I seek You; my soul thirsts for You; my flesh faints for You, as in a dry and weary land where there is no water. So I have looked for You. (Psalm 63:1-4)

> But from there you will seek the LORD your God and you will find Him, if you search after Him with all your heart and with all your soul. (Deuteronomy 4:29)

> The LORD looks down from heaven on the children of man, to see if there are any who understand, who seek after God. (Psalm 14:2)

> Wondrously show Your steadfast love, O Savior of those who seek refuge from their adversaries at Your right hand. (Psalm 17:7)

The afflicted shall eat and be satisfied; those who seek Him shall praise the LORD! May your hearts live forever! (Psalm 22:26)

Who shall ascend the hill of the LORD? And who shall stand in His holy place? He who has clean hands and a pure heart, who does not lift up his soul to what is false and does not swear deceitfully. He will receive a blessing from the LORD and righteousness from the God of his salvation. (Psalm 24:3-5)

One thing have I asked of the Lord, that will I seek after: that I may dwell in the house of the Lord all the days of my life, to gaze upon the beauty of the Lord and to inquire in his temple. (Psalm 27:4)

When You said, "Seek My face," my heart said to You, "Your face, O Lord, I shall seek. (Psalm 27:8) "

The young lions suffer want and hunger; but those who seek the LORD lack no good thing. (Psalm 34:10)

But may all who seek You rejoice and be glad in You; may those who love your salvation say continually, "Great is the LORD! (Psalm 40:16) "

O God, You are my God; earnestly I seek You; my soul thirsts for You; my flesh faints for You; as in a dry and weary land where there is no water. So I have looked upon You in Your sanctuary, beholding Your power and glory. Because Your steadfast love is better than life, my lips will praise You. So I will bless You as long as I live; in Your name I lift up my hands. My soul will be satisfied as with fat and rich food, and my mouth will praise You with joyful lips, when I remember You on upon my bed, and meditate on You in the watches of the night; for You have been my help, and in the shadow of Your wings I will sing for joy. (Psalm 63:1-7)

Seek the Lord and his strength; seek his presence continually! (Psalm 105:4)

Blessed are those who keep his testimonies, who seek him with their whole heart. (Psalm 119:2)

I love those who love Me, and those who seek Me diligently find Me. (Proverbs 8:17)

Many seek the face of a ruler, but it is from the Lord that a man gets justice. (Proverbs 29:26)

The path of the righteous is level; You make level the way of the righteous. In the path of Your judgments, O Lord, we wait for You; your name and remembrance are the desire of our soul. My soul yearns for You in the night; my spirit within me earnestly seeks You. For when Your judgments are in the earth, the inhabitants of the world learn righteousness. (Isaiah 26:7-9)

Seek the LORD while He may be found; call upon Him while He is near; let the wicked forsake his way, and the unrighteous man his thoughts; let him return to the LORD, that He may have compassion on him, and to our God, for He will abundantly pardon. For My thoughts are not your thoughts, neither are your ways My ways, declares the LORD. For as the heavens are higher than the earth, so are My ways higher than your ways and My thoughts than your thoughts. (Isaiah 55:6-9)

For I know the plans I have for you, declares the LORD, plans for welfare and not for evil, to give you a future and a hope. Then you will call upon Me and come and pray to Me, and I will hear you. You will seek Me and find Me, when you seek Me with all your heart. I will be found by you, declares the LORD, and I will restore your fortunes and gather you from all the nations and all the places where I have driven you, declares the LORD, and I will bring your back to the place from which I sent you into exile. (Jeremiah 29:1-14)

For the Gentiles seek after all these things (those who don't know God worry for and seek after material comforts and wealth), and your heavenly Father knows that you need them all. But seek first the kingdom of God and His righteousness, and all these things will be added to you. (Matthew 6:32-33; my explanation added)

Ask, and it will be given to you; seek, and you will find; knock, and it will be opened to you. For everyone who asks receives, and the one who seeks finds, and to the one who knocks it will be opened. Or which one of you, if his son asks him for bread, will give him a stone? Or if he asks for a fish, will give him a serpent? If you then, who are evil, know how to give good gifts to your children, how much more will your Father who is in heaven give good things to those who ask Him! (Matthew 7:7-11) "

If then you have been raised with Christ, seek the things that are above, where Christ is, seated at the right hand of God. (Colossians 3:1)

And without faith it is impossible to please Him, for whoever would draw near to God must believe that He exists and that He rewards those who seek Him. (Hebrews 11:6)

Just look at what God is saying to us! What a faith-building, hope-inspiring, peace-giving study of the blessing and profound privileges of walking with God. This is true happiness. This is true fulfillment. And this is free! I think this list is worth re-reading on a regular basis!

Make a short list of the blessings that speak most to you—and remember we just scratched the surface of the awesome reward of knowing God!

_____

_____

_____

_____

_____

_____

_____

_____

This is the right place to pause and thank God (an aspect of worship). Go to Him now and tell Him which promises mean the most to you and ask Him to lead you to Himself. He has already begun the process. He has placed you in this study of His Biblical Prescriptions for Life. Remember to thank Him for that, too.

WRAPPING IT UP

Do you want to seek God? Do you desire to know Him and experience His love and personhood more than anything else? If so, you're in good company. You, like King David, have a heart after God.

The study of "seeking" would be incomplete if we didn't wrap up with the most important seeking that will ever happen. That's because God Himself seeks us—and He always finds us! Want proof?

> Now the tax collectors and sinners were all drawing near to hear him. And the Pharisees and the scribes grumbled, saying, "This man receives sinners and eats with them." So he told them this parable: "What man of you, having a hundred sheep, if he has lost one of them, does not leave the ninety-nine in the open country, and go after the one that is lost, until he finds it? And when he has found it, he lays it on his shoulders, rejoicing. And when he comes home, he calls together his friends and his neighbors, saying to them, 'Rejoice with me, for I have found my sheep that was lost.' Just so, I tell you, there will be more joy in heaven over one sinner who repents than over ninety-nine righteous persons who need no repentance. (Luke 15:1-10)"
>
> For the Son of Man came to seek and to save the lost. (Luke 19:10)

Thank You, Father—the Good Shepherd—for seeking and finding me!

LIVING IN COMMUNITY

Share your story of how God found you with your study buddy today. Then ask them for their story. What an awesome, loving, relentlessly pursuing God we have!

BEING ON MISSION

Do you think there's someone you know who is beyond God's reach? The Bible says *no one* is beyond His reach. This would be a good day to start praying for that person consistently—that God would seek and draw him or her unto Himself, and that they would surrender to the Good Shepherd and come for healing by the Ultimate Physician.

COMMITMENT

Just one more day of study this week, one more day to put into practice your new Biblical Prescriptions for Life. If you've missed a day or more, don't be too hard on yourself. Instead, remember His mercies are new every morning. That includes *this* morning! Start now. Move forward on the path toward healing and whole-life, life-long wellness.

Every day this week, I've given you a dual walking/movement task. Today I want you to observe and listen. Listen for God's voice. Observe how He works in your life and around you. Have you noticed that when you move the body as well as the brain, the benefits increase? When we, with our hand in God's, heed the physical laws of the universe, there are spiritual benefits; and vice versa! Make movement and listening to God fun. Write in this weeks' movement journal how you can have more fun as you increase your movement. Walking while laughing, give it a try!

DAY 7

Your Day of Rest

Seek God today. He is moving toward you. Move toward Him as you answer these questions:

*   How did you experience His love toward you today? _____

*   How did you experience the movement of the walk of life as you moved toward Him?

    _____

*   Did the physical movement remind you of the spiritual movement? _____

This would be a great day to walk with God in worship, in nature, and with a friend in community. Use this space to record notes about today's Sabbath.

*   How did you invest it? _____

*   Where did you rest? _____

*   Did you join others in their rest? _____

*   Did you serve someone in an act of selfless love? _____

*   Did you spend some time in physical light? How did it feel? _____

*   What did you learn about God today? _____

Take some time to think about others who've walked with God: Enoch, Noah, Daniel, Moses, David, John the Baptist, and others. Sometime soon, take a few moments and study how they walked with God and determine what can be learned from them.

*   What did you learn about yourself today? _____

*   Did the people you have been praying for come to your mind spontaneously? _____

*   Did you pray for them again? _____

As you rest, take some time to breathe deeply and slowly. Now in all honesty answer these questions.

As you rest, remember the importance of rest, physical, mentally, and spiritually, to the body. Take some time to briefly think about the big picture items presented in the preceding lessons. Is God speaking to you?

Are you taking the time to hear His voice?

As you acknowledge Him as the healer, drink water, enjoy light, and move daily, are you feeling better? Do you feel empowered by your Creator?

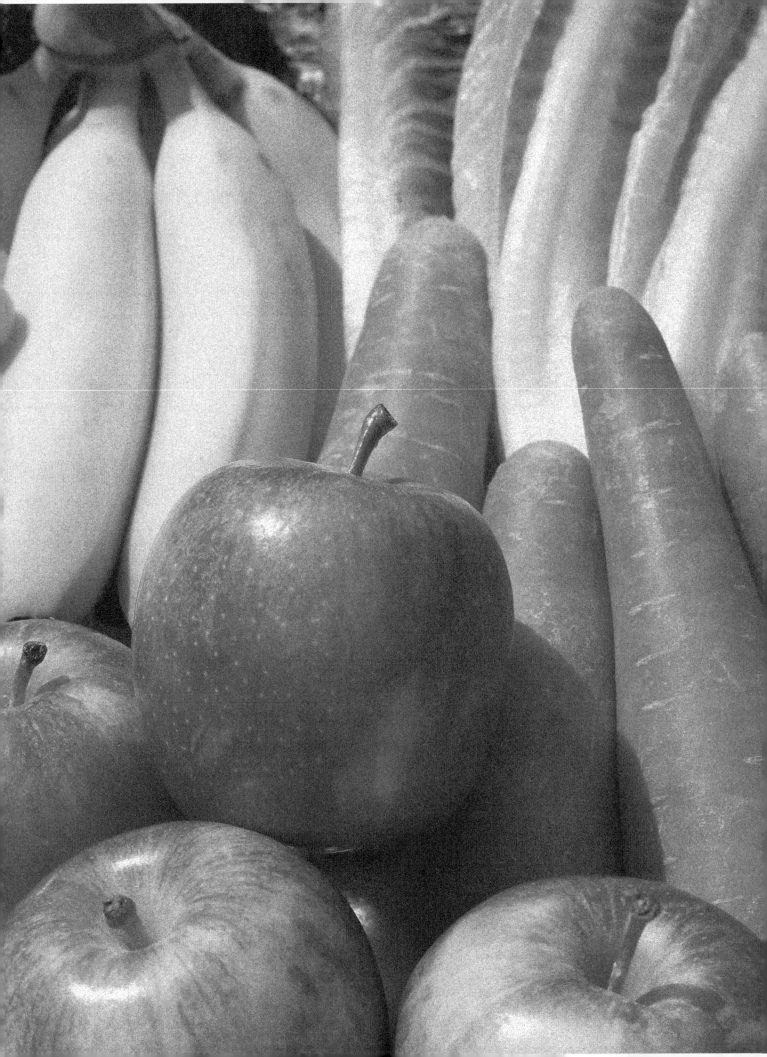

WEEK 5

Biblical Prescription for Life 4 — An Apple a Day

Kara has lived with type 1 diabetes since the age of 7. She was referred for follow-up after a stress test showed her heart was not receiving enough blood when she exerted herself. Angiography revealed many severe blockages in small arteries supplying blood to the heart. A cardiovascular surgeon, as well as two very experienced interventional cardiologists had evaluated her. All of them felt her arteries were too small for the placement of stents or bypass surgery.

Kara decided to get another opinion. Again, after careful evaluation, the new set of physicians concluded that procedures would not help her symptoms or chance of survival and, in fact, would likely make the situation worse. When she arrived for yet another opinion, she was more than discouraged and couldn't walk far before having symptoms. There just wasn't enough energy-supplying blood flowing throughout her heart. She understood that diabetes was tough on all arteries.

We began focusing on the positives. We examined causes of disease, the genetics, the nutrition, the stressors, and yes, the brain, and how her beliefs—along with all these other factors—affect her brain and ultimately the physiology. We talked about the complexities of the human body and how science and technology has yet to unwrap all the inner- workings of this wonderful created gift. I also reassured her that just because a symptom couldn't be treated with further procedures didn't mean we couldn't improve the symptoms and change the course of her physiology.

Today, three years later, Kara is doing well. She's living a full life without symptoms. At 46, she feels in control of her medical situation. How did she do it? The answer is really very simple. Much of her treatment has been focused on nutrition and avoiding the substance that was clogging her arteries—fat. She exercises 45 minutes to an hour daily and minimizes stress. This includes worship.

You've heard the old adage: An apple a day keeps the doctor away. There's an incredible amount of truth in that statement. Of course, Kara is doing more than eating an apple a day. When I asked if I could share her story in this series, she readily agreed and said, "Be sure to tell everyone to take one step at a time and remember the importance of spiritual food."

Are you ready to continue to take yet another step toward better health? This week we will begin on the path to improve your nutrition with both physical and spiritual food.

During the upcoming days we will introduce another Biblical Prescription. This treatment is one of the most powerful tools you have at your disposal to address a dizzying array of ailments and diseases. Scientists are almost tripping over themselves these days discovering just how powerful certain foods are at stopping and, in many cases, actually reversing some of our most concerning medical conditions.

Just how effective is nutrition when it comes to health? Nutrition is one of the ways to prevent and reverse chronic disease. That's right. We could reduce doctor visits, surgeries, premature deaths, and a whole lot of pain and suffering by simply changing what we eat. Most of our medical expense and about eighty percent of all doctor visits involve chronic disease. Proper nutrition, along with God's help, has the potential to address the cause of many chronic conditions from obesity and mental health problems to hypertension, diabetes and heart disease.

Yes, what we feed our body makes a huge difference. The often quoted "We are what we eat" has a lot of truth buried in it. What we put in our bodies carries consequences. The same can be said for the minds: inputs alter chemistry.

This week, be brutally honest with yourself. Do you choose to eat healthily? Are you putting high quality products into your body—and your mind? What are the steps—the baby steps—needed to improve both at the same time? We're going to find out!

As always, there needs to be a little mental preparation before beginning a journey of this importance. Keep in mind that God created us and knows all about our needs. That's why, right along with us, He created a world that could sustain our health at absolute optimum levels. Nothing was left out. He originally set us up to live forever with Him.

Sin put an end to that, but the pathways to health remain viable. Nutrition is one of those pathways we ignore at our own peril. You have had successes so far as we have studied together. Changing the way we eat is a journey as well. We must take the steps slowly. Some of this journey will move quickly while others will need more time. Let's support each other and pray for each other as we learn about and change our nutrition this week,

We must continue to open our minds to God's leading this week. Let's pray together. Feel free to use your own words, but your prayer might sound something like this:

Dear God, I need your help. I want to improve my nutrition, and take another step toward improving the body You lent me. Please help me as I learn more Biblical prescriptions for Life. Be with my study buddy and all the members of my group as we make this journey together. Thank you. Amen.

VIDEO GUIDE 5

Nutrition

VIDEO (20 minutes)

Major Bible verses:

•   Genesis: 1:29, 30

•   Daniel 1:12-20

•   Exodus 16:35

Write down a time in your life when you felt discouraged about your nutrition. _____

What do you think was making you discouraged? _____

According to our verses this week, what comprised the original diet? _____

Who was this diet designed for? _____

How long did it take Daniel's captors until they saw a difference in his health? _____

What was the magnitude of difference as recorded in Daniel 12:20? _____

Why did the Israelites need something from God to sustain them? _____

The video mentioned sources of energy. Do you remember what they are? _____

_____

Is it possible that your food choices are putting stress on your body? Explain _____

What is the Biblical Prescription for Life for week 5? _____

As a review, write down some of the Biblical Prescriptions for Life you are applying to your life:

1.   _____

2.   _____

3.   _____

4.   _____

Group discussion (20 minutes)

- After watching the video and listening to Kara's story, what do you think should be your first step in making nutritional changes?

- Is this step doable and how is it doable?

- What are potential roadblocks?

- How can you help each other attain these goals?

- How can you be a potential roadblock to someone trying to make changes?

- How can you be a potential roadblock to yourself as you try to make changes?

- What is the real key to make changes?

LIVING IN COMMUNITY

Daniel had friends who helped him in his journey. Likewise we have a group of friends who want to help this week. Take a moment after today's meeting to connect with at least one person. This week, call, email, or text this friend and share encouragement as changes is made. Do not be discouraged if you slip and slide a little as you make changes. Be sure to offer lots of praise over victories won!

INDIVIDUAL REFLECTION

You can be an effective provider for your own health and the good news is that the Ultimate Physician is there to assist you. That's right. The God of the Universe is scrubbed in and standing by your side, ready to guide your hands—and your mind—through the process of gaining and maintaining optimum health.

He may do this through reading the Bible, a thought, an impression, a statement made by a trusted friend, a video (like the one you just enjoyed), lines in a book, or simply the realization of truth. Our job is to listen and watch for His leading.

Remember Elijah in the cave? First there was the wind, then the earthquake, then the fire. But, according to 1 Kings chapter 19 verses through 13, God wasn't in those things. Next came the "still, small voice" and that's where Elijah finally heard the divine instructions he needed to hear. Listen for that still, small voice this week.

Make a short list of some of the changes you desire to make with God's help in regards to nutrition.

1. _____

2. _____

3. _____

4. _____

As simple changes are made, you will feel better as your physiology improves and the next change will be easier. As you realize the impact of these changes, you will want to continue to improve your nutrition. When eating poorly causes a noticeable change in the way you feel and think, it will be even easier to continue finding practical ways to improve your nutrition.

BEING MISSIONAL

Would you like to share your newfound information concerning building and maintaining optimum health? Here's a suggestion. Don't become a health evangelist and start "preaching" at work or at home. This approach may turn some away. Instead, starting *living* the truth you're learning. Let them see the changes taking place in your life without you having to point them out. Trust me, as you follow the Biblical Prescriptions for Life, there will be changes both in you physically (less weight, more energy) and spiritually (less sadness, more gladness). Start by committing this verse to memory:

> Let your light so shine before men [and women], that they may see your good works, and glorify your Father, which is in heaven (Matthew 5:16).

Notice the last part of that verse. Who should get all the praise when people see changes in you?

_____

_____

Write down several ideas of how you can be lovingly share the information you've learned so far: _____

_____

_____

_____

COMMITMENT

"This week, I am going to ADD and DO at least one of the following simple Biblical Prescriptions for Life:"

I commit to	Biblical Prescriptions for Life	Day 1	2	3	4	5	6	7
	Read aloud 5x each day. Practice, memorize & recite:							
	Genesis 1:29-30 "And God said, 'Behold, I have given you every plant yielding seed that is on the face of the earth, and every tree with seed in its fruit. You shall have them for food. And to every beast of the earth and to every bird of the heavens and to every-thing that creeps on the earth, everything that has the breath of life, I have given every green plant for food.' And so it does"							

	Daniel 1:12-13 *"Test your servants for ten days; let us be given vegetables to eat and water to drink, Then let our appearance and the appearance of the youths who eat the king's food be observed by you, and deal with your servants according to what you see."*							
	Journal my food choices and eating habits for the week.							
	Add one cup of leafy greens to my mid-day and evening meal each day.							
	Add 3-5 servings of fresh fruits and vegetables to my diet each day.							
	Reduce my use of refined sugar by half each day.							
	Reduce my consumption of meat by 30% this week.							
	Make breakfast the biggest meal of the day and dinner the smallest.							

If you missed a session or want to review one, go to biblicalprescriptionsforlife.com to stream Dr. Marcum's audio and video.

DAY 1

Why Nutrition?

Let's start off today's lesson by reviewing the Biblical Prescription for Life found in Genesis. Remember, Genesis contains the Creation story and reveals to us a wonderful truth. God not only created us, He created all that we'd need to stay healthy *forever*. It was all there in the Garden of Eden in perfect, pristine condition!

Read Genesis 1:29, 30:

> And God said, "See, I have given you every herb that yields seed which is on the face of all the earth, and every tree whose fruit yields seed; to you it shall be for food. Also, to every beast of the earth, to every bird of the air, and everything that creeps on the on earth, in which there is life, I have given every green herb for food"; and it was so.

On the sixth day of creation, God not only made Adam and Eve, He also provided His personal nutritional guidelines and recommendations. It was for a whole-food, plant-based diet. The original diet was very fresh, very available, and very *green*. Nowhere do we find a list of fast or processed foods. Nutrition was a gift built into the plants that filled the garden home. The plants had the nutritional components in the correct ratios to promote optimal health. Why is this so important today? Why are we just now, as a society, emphasizing nutrition?

I look at our mindset towards health today and I cringe. Every year, the rate of heart attacks, strokes, cancer, dementia, osteoporosis, diabetes, sleep apnea, obesity, joint problems, and mental health disease continue to rise. Yet, at the very same time, prescription medicine usage is at an all time high. More and more people are needing care. The evidence is conclusive as far as I'm concerned. Modern medicine is great at treating acute problems such as heart attacks, bacterial infections, a slow heart rate, or a broken arm. But for *chronic* disease—those ailments that seem to take up residence in our bodies and just stay there year after painful year—modern medicine falls short. It's great at treating symptoms but as I have said before, often does not address the cause, the original stressor. Also, in the background, shrouded by the false sense of security that comes with a reduction of symptoms, the stressor continues its persistent and extremely damaging rampage.

But that's just the tip of the iceberg. It doesn't take very long to figure out that the current system of treating symptoms is unsustainable. It might keep the pharmaceutical, health-care, and insurance industries busy, but is not fixing the problem. Someday, society is going to wake up and say, "Hey, this isn't working." I believe that realization is already starting to take hold and I'm glad. Be honest with yourself. Look at the evidence in the world. Is our current system working? Is change needed? How can these changes be enacted?

As technology has improved, we've moved away from the original plan that God put in place six thousand years ago. This has put a tremendous stress on the body. Contrary to what the drug companies want us to believe, easier is not always better. A pill for every ill isn't working. As a matter of fact, it's making things worse.

Even the culture in which we live doesn't promote healthy nutrition. We want it easy here, too. We want it fast, over-the-top tasty, and have the shelf life of a rock. But I keep coming back to that statement: We are what we eat! Our bodies were created to run best on a plant-based diet. As we'll learn this week, the benefits are beyond amazing.

In Bible times, they weren't faced with some of the problems we have. Yes, many didn't have enough food to eat. It's the same today; food insecurity is still a global problem. But hear me out: in some places, more people die of overeating than undereating. Consider these statistics offered by the World Health Organization (*Fact Sheet N-311, January, 2015*):

- Worldwide obesity has more than doubled since 1980.

- In 2014, more than 1.9 billion adults, 18 years and older, were overweight. Of these over 600 million were obese.

- 39% of adults aged 18 years and over were overweight in 2014, and 13% were obese.

- Most of the world's population lives in countries where overweight and obesity kills more people than underweight.

- 42 million children under the age of 5 were overweight or obese in 2013.

- Obesity is largely preventable.

It's tragic that in a land filled with food, people are eating themselves to death.

Thank God that it doesn't have to be this way! Our Creator has given us sound, scientifically proven advice on how to keep ourselves—and those we love—healthy. His words are timeless as if He knew we'd need this prescription.

This week, we'll discover the importance of good nutrition and try to apply some healthy changes into our lives one-step at a time. Some of you will be hearing about this for the first time. For others, it will provide a handy review. But we'll all be learning how plant-based nutrition changes the entire body and not just one chemical pathway. God has given us a powerful prescription for health in the plants He created.

How is this accomplished? The sun supplies energy to the earth. Plants take sunlight and carbon dioxide and transform them into oxygen and food. We have the opportunity to eat our energy supply first-hand! It doesn't have to pass through the body of an animal, where most of it is used up. It doesn't have to be processed out in a factory as various chemicals and preservatives are added. We can enjoy God's bounty right out of the ground or right from the branches of a living tree.

We will discover this week the incredible healing benefits of plants and the spiritual benefits of eating plants. Yes, *spiritual* benefits! I invite you to have an open mind as we learn about nutrition.

Look at the text for today once more. Read it slowly and thoughtfully. God has given us a gift. Our Heavenly Father wants the best for His children and, to provide it, He's not going to give us any junk. His recommendation on nutrition applies more than ever in today's world.

And don't think for a minute that God saved the best just for this world. He is also planning to reestablish the Eden-like ideal in the Earth Made New! Read the following passages and:

- Circle words that describe a condition found on this earth.
- Place a box around words that do NOT describe a condition found on this earth.

They shall not hurt or destroy in all My holy mountain; for the earth shall be full of the knowledge of the Lord as the waters cover the sea. (Isaiah 11:9)

Then the angel showed me the river of the water of life, bright as crystal, flowing from the throne of God and of the Lamb 2 through the middle of the street of the city; also, on either side of the river, the tree of life with its twelve kinds of fruit, yielding its fruit each month. The leaves of the tree were for the healing of the nations. \\\

No longer will there be anything accursed, but the throne of God and of the Lamb will be in it, and his servants will worship him. They will see his face, and his name will be on their foreheads. And night will be no more.

They will need no light of lamp or sun, for the Lord God will be their light, and they will reign forever and ever. (Revelation 22:1-5)

Heaven sounds pretty good to me! How does it sound to you? Write here what attracts you most about this *Earth Made New* God is preparing for us all. _____

List three ways we can at least attempt to bring this old world a little closer to Heaven's ideal:

1. _____

2. _____

3. _____

Where do you see what we eat fitting in to that ideal: _____

Are you beginning to see any connections between physical nutrition and spiritual nutrition? Write it down here:

_____

So far in our study, we've discovered that God doesn't do anything unless:

- It's good for us.

- It's good for those around us.

- It's good for the earth.

Sin, on the other hand, is just the opposite. From your own experience, write down how you think the devil has taken something good from God and twisted it around to be harmful:

- God made _____ good for us, but the devil turned it into _____ that is bad for us.

- God made _____ good for those around us, but the devil turned it into _____ that is bad for those around us.

- God made _____ good for the earth, but the devil turned in into _____ that is bad for the earth.

When it comes to nutrition, we face the very same question Adam and Eve faced: Whom are you going to believe? Who are you going to trust? Who are you going to follow with your worship? It's my goal to turn your attention to God's timeless truth. Doing so can make you both physically and spiritually healthy!

WRAPPING IT UP

If you wanted expert advice, where would you turn? Would you believe the advertisements, the Internet, or commercials? Do they want what's best for you or is their goal to sell you a product? There is a reason that the world is so sick. Genetics, nutrition, environmental inputs, and our brains determine our health. We can't change our genes, but we can certainly change the way genetics are expressed with our nutrition and our brains.

LIVING IN COMMUNITY

Plan a time when you can go to a fast food restaurant and just observe how your response to that environment has changed. Write down your observations and share them with the group this week. Do this again at the end of the week and compare your notes. How have your feelings about what you're seeing changed over time?

This week, be positive and remember to love and not judge others. Everyone is moving at different speeds. We need to be supportive, even when it comes to food choices. This is a journey.

BEING MISSIONAL

What did God impress you with from the verses in Genesis? Talk to your study buddy about how you can continue to encourage one another. This week is a little different from our preceding weeks. Hopefully, others will see the changes in your life and ask you about them. Your example will help others.

COMMITMENT

Remember the lessons on water? Water is at the foundation of good nutrition. You have already started on the path to better nutrition just by drinking enough water—plant-based foods are 70% water.

Take a moment to review the lessons on water. As we move through the week, I am going to ask you to commit to doing something each day. Today, I want you to focus on drinking more water if you're still behind the curve on this Biblical Prescription.

Let's start to journal the food we are eating. I encourage you to write down everything you eat this week. This includes snacks, restaurant foods, *everything* you put in your mouth. This can be private and will give you a good indication of the types of foods you consume regularly.

Day 1:

Breakfast _____

Lunch _____

Dinner _____

Day 2:

Breakfast _____

Lunch _____

Dinner _____

Day 3:

Breakfast _____

Lunch _____

Dinner _____

Day 4:

Breakfast _____

Lunch _____

Dinner _____

Day 5:

Breakfast _____

Lunch _____

Dinner _____

Day 6

Breakfast _____

Lunch _____

Dinner _____

Day 7:

Breakfast _____

Lunch _____

Dinner _____

— DAY 2 —

Lessons from China

When patients return with the same health problems over and over again, I search for answers. It didn't take long to realize that the best healing textbook was the Bible! After all, God the Creator—the One who designed the earth from the ground up to support human life—should have the perfect understanding on what human life needs to thrive. Within the pages of the Bible are divine prescriptions, recommendations, counsel, that I can offer patients. There is also evidence from studies to support these Biblical Prescriptions. Modern medicine has made great advances especially for acute problems and in helping alleviate the stress of poor genetics. As the science of Biblical Prescriptions has progressed, there is now something more to offer—treatments with few, if any, side effects, and very little cost, treatments that address symptoms and cause. An individual patient should always look at the evidence and decide on the various treatments based on the associated risk/benefit profile.

According to Bible study, prayer and scientific literature, treatments such as water, movement, nutrition, light, rest and fresh air can be used as powerful prescriptions, capable of delivering healing as well as preventing physical problems. Again let me emphasize, these treatments are capable of addressing cause rather than merely dealing with a symptom.

Being a scientist both at heart and by vocation, I have turned to science for proof and have not been disappointed. The evidence is not only there, it is being reaffirmed on an almost daily basis. I can't tell you how exciting it is to have the tools at my disposal to prevent and treat disease! With the help of Biblical Prescriptions, I have the opportunity to help my patients beyond treating symptoms. I can bring them face-to-face with the causes of their ailments. If you remove the cause, you've cured the patient. All that was needed were the "right" tools.

As I mentioned, I discovered that the treatment for many chronic diseases was the food we eat. God gave the original recommendations we read about in Genesis. Scientific proof was found from a surprising place: rural China.

In the groundbreaking book, "The China Study" released in 2006, T. Colin Campbell presented the most comprehensive study of nutrition ever performed. A team of researchers, headed by nutritionalist/epidemiologist Campbell traveled to China to study the relationship between diet and disease. They interviewed and studied the records of over 6,000 individuals. The results surprised even the scientists. Their findings provided repeatable scientific evidence that an animal-based diet causes disease. They also found conclusive evidence that a plant-based diet *heals* disease. When I finished reading the last chapter and silently closed the book, I knew I now had the strongest scientific proof for God's recommendations in Genesis.

Over the years, I have had the privilege to become friends with Dr. Campbell. He has appeared on the television program "Heart of Health Live," and been a frequent guest on our radio program, "Heartwise with Charles Mills." When he and his son, Nelson, asked me to help promote his latest movie, *Plant Pure Nation*, I agreed immediately! Through his evidence-based research, Dr. Campbell has proven that diets made up mostly of animal products cause disease while eating more plants is a proven way to prevent and treat disease. I strongly recommend that you add *The China Study* to your library. Just the first 100 pages will change your life! Also take a look at the films, *Forks over Knives* and *PlantPure Nation*. They will inspire you in your steps toward improved nutrition.

Since writing the book, Dr. Campbell has been travelling the world promoting this plant-centered message as a way to improve health, change the economy, and save our environment. But you and I now know that God gave us this prescription at the very beginning of earth's history. So why does the public not know about this? Why are current, governmental dietary guidelines lacking these insights? Why does the general public not know the truth? Why are physicians not touting nutrition to a greater degree?

There is some good news and some bad news. First, the bad: Nutrition isn't being taught to doctors on an appropriate scale in medical school, Your provider may not have the needed education to promote proper nutrition. Now, the good news: that's changing! More and more doctors, especially young, up-and-coming professionals, are more attuned to the evidence from the latest scientific research. They're much more likely to say, "In order to avoid another heart attack (or recurrence of cancer, or development of dementia), you need to turn to a plant-based diet as advocated and proven in *The China Study*. The ones who've done their homework will also add, "'This isn't necessarily being a vegetarian, as some vegetarians can still consume oil-, salt-, and sugar-filled junk. You just need to eat as much whole plant foods as you can.'"

Some call plant-based nutrition "extreme." Our Creator and Master Designer didn't think this was extreme, but designed it to be the norm. Having a breastbone sawed in two to perform a bypass of fat-clogged arteries, or having a breast, prostate, colon, lung or other body part removed because of cancer—now that's extreme. That said, there does seem to be resistance from the general public concerning food choices. Bad habits are hard to break. But the tide is turning here as well as people are getting sick and tired of being sick and tired. They're also tired of knowing that nearly one in five of their hard-earned dollars are being spent on a healthcare program that promotes the treatment of symptoms. They want to get well while they protect the environment from the dangerous greenhouse gasses generated by the meat processing industry.

We must know and apply the truth! Why? I'll let the Bible answer that question. Read and then write out—word for word—this exciting text:

> So Jesus said to the Jews who had believed him, "If you abide in my word, you are truly my disciples, and you will know the truth, and the truth will set you free. (John 8:31, 32)"

_____

_____

These are truly life-changing words. If I hold to God's teachings—if I embrace God's design for health and well-being and share His Biblical Prescriptions for Life--God can set me free from so many of today's common illnesses and use me to help others. We can be free of diabetes, heart disease, high blood pressure, atherosclerosis, osteoporosis, obesity, many cancers, and on and on and on.

Each of you is learning new truth this week and will have some new steps to take. I want to finish today with a text that has always helped me. We memorized this text in week one.

> Come to me, all who labor and are heavy laden, and I will give you rest. Take my yoke upon you, and learn from me, for I am gentle and lowly in heart, and you will find rest for your souls. For my yoke is easy, and my burden is light. (Matthew 11:28-30)

Take a moment to write the text above on a piece of paper or small card and place it where you'll see it every day this week. Remember, my friend T. Colin Campbell didn't originate the whole food, plant-based diet. He simply documented its incredible power to fight disease and heal the human body. It was God, our Creator, who lovingly placed all that power in plants, and then made them available to all who would "hold to my teaching."

WRAPPING IT UP

As we're learning about the plant-based diet, take some time to do some research on your own. Look back at groups of healthy people: rural China, Okinawa, or Norway during World War 2. Do they (or did they) suffer from chronic diseases like heart disease, diabetes, hypertension, cancer, and mental health problems? What do these areas have in common?

LIVING IN COMMUNITY

Take some time now to right down three healthy places where you can eat out. These restaurants would need to provide items from the plant world like great salads, fiber-rich grains, yummy beans, and lots of raw fruits.

1. _____

2. _____

3. _____

Share this information with the group. Also, don't forget to encourage each member and the new friendships you've been developing during this study.

Now, we can go on a walk with a friend in the sunlight while drinking water and eating a fresh apple while saying a prayer of thanksgiving and know beyond doubt that you're applying Biblical Prescriptions for Life!

BEING MISSIONAL

As you learn about nutrition, what are some simple steps you can suggest to those who ask you about nutrition? Notice I said "those who ask." Nutrition is very personal and must be approached in a loving, not judging, one-step-at-a-time manner. Keep in mind the old adage for writers: don't tell, *show*.

COMMITMENT

Today I want you to commit to your food diary. Yesterday, you focused on drinking water. Now, start making the evening meal your smallest one and enjoy it a little earlier. This will give your digestive track more time to rest. Get up tomorrow and "break the fast" by eating your biggest meal in the morning. How about a big bowl of oatmeal with walnuts, fresh berries, and a tall glass of cool water? Document how you feel after making this important step to improve your nutrition.

Continue to pray for God's guidance in your life. Remember, He's standing by your side.

— DAY 3 —

Dan the Man

So far this week, we've seen in Kara how good nutrition changes the body. We discovered in Genesis God's original nutritional recommendations and were introduced to the concept of a plant-based diet. I want to start today's lesson with another of my favorite stories from the book of Daniel.

Daniel was a young man when he was forcibly relocated to Babylon in 605 B. C. He'd been raised in a good Judean home and was, as the Bible describes, "without blemish." When Daniel, along with some other similar young people, was selected to receive special favors from Nebuchadnezzar, King of Babylon, a Biblical Prescription for Life emerged. Let's read the story as recorded in Daniel 1:8-20:

> But Daniel resolved that he would not defile himself with the king's food, or with the wine that he drank. Therefore he asked the chief of the eunuchs to allow him not to defile himself.
>
> And God gave Daniel favor and compassion in the sight of the chief of the eunuchs, and the chief of the eunuchs said to Daniel, "I fear my lord the king, who assigned your food and your drink; for why should he see that you were in worse condition than the youths who are of your own age? So you would endanger my head with the king."
>
> Then Daniel said to the steward whom the chief of the eunuchs had assigned over Daniel, Hananiah, Mishael, and Azariah, "Test your servants for ten days; let us be given vegetables to eat and water to drink. Then let our appearance and the appearance of the youths who eat the king's food be observed by you, and deal with your servants according to what you see." So he listened to them in this matter, and tested them for ten days.
>
> At the end of ten days it was seen that they were better in appearance and fatter in flesh than all the youths who ate the king's food. So the steward took away their food and the wine they were to drink, and gave them vegetables.
>
> As for these four youths, God gave them learning and skill in all literature and wisdom, and Daniel had understanding in all visions and dreams.
>
> At the end of the time, when the king had commanded that they should be brought in, the chief of the eunuchs brought them in before Nebuchadnezzar. And the king spoke with them, and among all of them none was found like Daniel, Hananiah, Mishael, and Azariah. Therefore they stood before the king. And in every matter of wisdom and understanding about which the king inquired of them, he found them ten times better than all the magicians and enchanters that were in all his kingdom. (Daniel 1:8-20)

Wow! What a story! Evidently Daniel had been trained regarding a plant-based diet by his parents. Now, here in Babylon, he found himself captive in a foreign land. Yet, he was willing to stand up for what he believed to be the truth. He and his three companions ate *zeroim*, "that which is sown." After just ten days, a difference in how they looked could be easily seen. But their health was much more than skin deep. At the end of their training, a tenfold difference was noted. No wonder the king wanted Daniel's expertise in managing the strongest empire on Earth at that time.

Are you seeing the connection with Eden in this story? Daniel, along with his friends, was blessed by following the Creator's advice. They were applying a Biblical Prescription countering the culture surrounding them and were blessed. They were blessed physically and mentally.

This reminds me of my car. When I picked it up at the dealer, it came with a small booklet tucked neatly in the glove compartment. In this booklet, I found carefully selected sets of rules and suggestions—all designed to make my new purchase last for miles and miles and miles. One of those rules stated that this particular automobile burns unleaded fuel.

What would you think if I merrily drove my car off the lot, stopped at a nearby gas station, and topped it off with diesel fuel, or propane, or kerosene? Hey, why not just dump water into the tank? It's cheaper and less work! If I did that, you'd point out that I wasn't following the owner's manual. Actually, my car would point out that fact even faster. How? It wouldn't start and, if it did, it wouldn't go very far. The statement "this automobile burns unleaded fuel" is there for a purpose.

Well, God, in His infinite love, handed Adam and Eve (and us) an owner's manual for our bodies. The first chapter of Genesis outlines, beyond a doubt, what we need to do to live optimally. However, if we ignore those rules and suggestions, we either will fail to start or will be greatly hindered in our journey. Cars need fuel. So do we. My car needs unleaded fuel. My body needs plants.

It may surprise you to know that you probably have a good supply of this all-important fuel in your pantry right now. Think about your store of food that's resting on your kitchen shelves or in your refrigerator at this very moment and write down "that which is sowed" i.e. plants or plant-based. Don't forget to include all your yummy fruits, seeds, and nuts, too:

_____

_____

_____

_____

_____

As we'll learn in lessons ahead, there are measurable changes in the brain that take place when we give our bodies the correct fuel. Topping off with fruits, vegetables, grains, seeds, and nuts doesn't create stress and inflammation. Instead, it enhances blood flow, lowers inflammation, and enhances our overall chemistry from proper bowel flora.

If I had the opportunity to examine Daniel and the king's men after that 10-day test, I know what I would find. I'm sure Daniel would present with a lower blood pressure, slower heart rate, less fat on and in his body, better sleep patterns, and was happier than the others. I'm sure his brainpower was off the chart.

And speaking of brainpower, this enhancement gave him an even greater ability to communicate with God. As we will learn in our final lesson, it was not only the food, but also the worship that changed his chemistry. And, yes, these types of changes are available to us as well.

Bottom line: Daniel followed truth to honor God, which also improved his chemistry.

Let's take a moment to review some of the things we've learned so far. Fill in the missing words of these texts to discover God's Health Principles mentioned in various parts of the Bible. They all have roots in the Creation story.

PROPER DIET: "And God said, "Behold, I have given you every _____ _____ _____ that is on the face of all the earth, and every _____ with _____ in its _____. You shall have them for _____. (Genesis 1:29)"

MOVEMENT: "He gives _____ to the faint, and to him who has no might he increases _____. (Isaiah 40:29)"

WATER: "Come, everyone who _____, come to the _____. (Isaiah 55:1)"

SUNSHINE: "Light is sweet, and it is pleasant for the eyes to see the sun. (Ecclesiastes 11:7)"

TEMPERANCE: "For this very reason, make every effort to supplement your faith with virtue, and virtue with knowledge, and knowledge with _____-_____. (2 Peter 15:6)"

REST: "Come to me, all who _____ and are _____ _____, and I will give you _____. (Matthew 11:28)"

WORSHIP: "The Lord helps them and delivers them; he delivers them from the wicked and saves them, because they _____ _____ in him. (Psalm 37:40)

LIVING IN COMMUNITY

Think about what has been the predominate food in communities throughout the ages. The Aztecs filled their stomachs with corn. The Incan empire lived basically on potatoes. The people of China enjoyed an abundance of rice. The Eastern world grew and ate grain.

Now think about what the predominate foods are today. In the modernized world, topping the shopping list are meats and processed foods. These "foods of the kings," rich in animal proteins, salts, fats, and sugar, are now available to the masses. But there's a dark side to this fact. With this change of nutrition has come the meteoric rise of acquired disease.

Take a poll in your study group. What is the main food source? Is it animal based or starch based (that which is grown or "sown"). Don't worry about the results. We're learning a much better way of eating—and living.

Also, take time this week to find a plant-based recipe to share with the group. Pick something that tastes good and that's easy to put together. If this goes well, your group just might develop a mini recipe book. Don't forget to send me a copy!

BEING MISSIONAL

One of the greatest ways to help our neighbors is by being a good example. What do you think the king's men were saying about Daniel before the test was completed? Do you think, if you stepped out like Daniel did, you'd receive a similar response from your neighbors? They may not know the truth as you know it. Their brains may have downshifted to selfishness and not love. Some may even feel threatened by your improved health and stamina. Just love them where they are and keep doing what you're doing. Dare to be a Daniel in today's world.

COMMITMENT

Today, I want you to try to eat 3 or more servings of fresh fruits and vegetables. Also consider a 10-day trial of just eating that which is sown. This might serve as a motivational moment because you'll begin to see how well your countenance improves after those ten days. If you are interested in this, go to the website plantpurenation.com or pcrm.org. These are great resources for those who want to move to optimum health faster.

Don't forget to:

- Drink water.

- Eat a big, hearty breakfast.

- Enjoy much smaller meals at night.

Today you are adding another step, at least 3 servings, hopefully more of fruits and vegetables.

Keep a list of your nutrition this week. Are you feeling better? If you find yourself hungrier eat a handful of almonds or walnuts. Celery or carrot sticks might help as well. Fiber is filling. We'll talk more about fiber tomorrow.

You're about to discover some of the many blessings in following Biblical Prescriptions for Life.

DAY 4

Food as Medicine

I met Melinda a few years ago after her doctor referred her to me for chest pain. She'd suffered from various ailments for years and had already received a diagnosis of fibromyalgia. As a busy home-schooling mom with three kids, she really didn't have time to deal with pain and was looking for answers. It was easy to see that my patient was open for a change—any change—that would improve her life.

Melinda enjoyed an active spiritual life and was constantly praying for healing. After a complete examination and a few confirmatory tests, I was convinced that her heart was just fine. So, what was the problem?

I asked about her nutrition. She hadn't really thought of this as a physical input which could be causing her any type of health problem. I carefully explained how our bodies are designed for a certain nutrient composition: 10-15% fat, 10-15% protein, and the rest carbohydrates—all of which are best served by plant-based sources. She seemed surprised, as she'd never heard these recommendations before.

"Just think about all the preservatives and chemicals we ingest and don't even know what they do," I told her. "Think about the chicken—made up of mostly fat and protein with no nutrients. Chicken feed is often laced with growth hormones, antibiotics (some animal antibiotics have contained arsenic), and disease-promoting chemicals. When our body sees this meal coming down our throats, our bowel flora is changed to fight what it considers to be an intruder. Our entire chemical makeup is altered. The fat is stored and much of the other material is sent circulating through our blood stream where it travels to every corner of our body. And that's just the beginning!"

Melinda agreed that what I just outlined didn't seem like a health-promoting way to nourish ourselves and asked if there was an alternative. I suggested she try going to a plant-based diet, just in case some of these chemicals were activating her immune system and triggering inflammation throughout her body. "I could never go plant-based," she lamented.

"Remember," I urged, "plant-based does not equal vegan or vegetarian. Plenty of foods that are technically vegan or vegetarian are refined and can contain overloads of salts, fats, and sugar. 'Plant-based' means that you focus on *whole foods* while staying positive and moving one step at a time." I also stated that eating this way for ten days was a great way to start. "You can do anything for ten days," I explained. "Aren't you tired of the pain?"

Melinda made the changes and her body responded. Over time, she has found ways to substitute the foods she thought she needed with the vast array of plants. With over twenty types of beans, various greens, berries, roots, and colorful fruits to round things out, she discovered that the plant kingdom offered much more variety than the animal kingdom ever did.

She still has an urge to return to the "Dark Side" occasionally. But, now, when she eats poorly, she feels poorly, so her new lifestyle has become self-regulating. Another benefit? She told me, "I actually never knew what feeling healthy was like. Now I do."

I recently had the opportunity to visit Dr. Caldwell Esselstyn at the Cleveland Clinic. His research has been revolutionary in cardiology and he's published studies documenting the actual reversal of heart disease with a plant-based diet. For those interested, his book, *Prevent and Reverse Heart Disease* is not only a best seller, but has helped many avoid a risky procedure to stabilize their heart disease. He refers to heart disease as a "paper tiger" and I totally agree.

Dr. Esselstyn uses food as medicine. In his book he describes the physiology of taking in too much fat. Too much fat paralyzes the important chemical nitric oxide, which helps regulate the health and flexibility of arteries of the heart and entire body. He shows how plants promote the formation of nitric oxide that, in turn, promotes the health of the endothelium—the lining of our blood vessels. The bottom line is: eat less fat and more greens and beans. The mechanisms behind how plants can be used as medicine are rapidly advancing, as people want safer ways to improve their bodies.

Another well-received health promoter, Dr. Michael Greger, has done much research into the area of clinical nutrition. His wildly popular website, *nutritionfacts.org*, should be on everyone's favorites list. Here he reviews all English-language evidence-based research and demonstrates how plants can change the chemistry of the entire body. I want to share some of this incredible, scientifically proven evidence with you:

- Cherries help fight gout and inflammation.

- Greens and beans can reduce angina and lower blood pressure. Improves energy use at the mitochondrial level.

- Beets lower blood pressure.

- Hibiscus tea lowers blood pressure.

- Ginger fights inflammation and migraines.

- Berries are powerful anti-oxidants and help prevent dementia and aging.

- Turmeric helps fight cancer and inflammation.

- Fiber lowers cholesterol and decreases the risk of cancer, improves bowel flora.

- Kiwi can help with infections.

- Strawberries can help with esophageal problems.

- Watermelons help revive sore muscles.

- Peppermint eases irritable bowel syndrome.

- Walnuts lower cardiovascular disease risk.

- Flax with lignands lowers the risk of breast cancer.

Dr. Greger, at his site, offers abundant references and reviews the evidence.

"Let food be thy medicine" - Hippocrates

97% of Americans get enough protein (Most comes from animal sources. Plant protein is a much safer source), and the 3% who do not, are usually on extreme caloric restriction. Now, pay close attention to this:

- 90+% of Americans are deficient in nutrients and fiber.

- 96% do not eat enough greens.

- 99% do not eat enough grains.

- Many don't know that exercise/movement improves nutrient absorption.

In one study I read recently, eating five fruits and veggies a day increase lifespan by three years! In a Taiwanese study, 50 cents a day spent on veggies lowered mortality by fifty percent.

90+% of Americans do not ingest enough fiber. This is a stressor. Fiber feeds the cells lining the colon. Short chain fatty acids are made. Butyrate is made which feeds the bowel. This helps absorption of electrolytes and regulates the trillion bacteria in the bowel. The bowel makes more of the good bacteria, which are involved, in many important chemical reactions. Without fiber, the bad bacteria have more influence on the physiology leading to inflammation and hindering the good bacteria.

Also attached to the fiber we ingest are polyphenols and phytonutrients. These chemical compounds serve as antioxidants and anti-inflammatory actions.

These reactions affect even our DNA repair mechanisms as well as aging. As time goes on we will learn more and more about the importance of fiber to the body.

I hope I've convinced you that food can serve as medicine. The studies have already been done. The results have already been tabulated. The evidence is overwhelming! More studies are on the way. What God put in place six thousand years ago in a beautiful garden called Eden is just as reliable and powerful today as it was then. By eating according to God's Health Plan, we can prevent untold problems and turn the tide on many of our acquired health problems. I call that very good news!

WRAPPING IT UP

In today's lesson, the take-home point is clear: food can be used as medicine especially for chronic disease. By eating well we can prevent many of the ailments plaguing this old world. There are *no side effects* and the long term benefits to the economy and ecology of the planet are significant.

LIVING IN COMMUNITY

Take some time to consider how you can make improvements in your own nutrition. Could you start by eating only plants one day a week? Two days a week? One meal a day? Give your friends a call and make sure they're still keeping their food diaries and looking for a healthy recipe to share with the group. Pray for each other daily.

BEING MISSIONAL

Christ met the needs of others and healing minds and bodies was one of His most effective tools. Healing can occur through lifestyle changes and through others—like you—whom God has blessed. Yes, you can be a healer. He also uses modern medicine to address the needs of the suffering. If God places you on a path of service this week, don't hesitate to share what you know. And, as always, continue to pray for our world.

COMMITMENT

Remember to take the time to visit the websites I mentioned. My own website, *heartwiseministries.org,* has many resources. Click on the "Radio" button and enjoy "Heartwise with Charles Mills." These 30-minute programs include interviews with health luminaries such as Caldwell Esselstyn, T. Colin Campbell, and Michael Greger. Charles' guests have much to say about nutrition and the power of food to help bring health to minds, bodies, and souls. If you're like me, you enjoy learning a little at a time. Then you can let your brain process that information and slowly apply what you've learned to how you live. Remember, health is a journey. But the sooner you start that journey, the sooner you'll reach your destination! Your group might want to expand and repeat the studies again.

By now, you have tried drinking water, eating breakfast, and eating earlier in the evening. Hopefully 3-5 fresh fruits and vegetables have been added to your daily diet.

Today, I want you to make yourself some healthy snacks! Try tossing some cut up veggies like carrots, celery, or greens in small zip lock bags to take with you to work or school. When hunger strikes, strike back with a healthy snack. Fruits like apples, oranges, and berries are good snacks as well. Feel free to include a few walnuts or almonds. If you make up an assortment of these "snack bags" and take them with you when you are out, you'll be much less tempted to visit a local fast-food restaurant or candy machine (neither of which were found in the Garden of Eden). Try this and report back.

— DAY 5 —————————————

Bread Alone?

If you take a few moments to think about what you've learned during the past few weeks, I hope you remember both the physical *and the spiritual* lessons. Today, the importance of linking the physical and the spiritual will be even more evident.

We've covered how stress changes the body chemistry whenever we move from God's original template for life to the modern substitute for life filled with fast foods, fast-lane living, and fast satisfactions. God's original plan also included a relationship with Him. When we emphasized the importance of water, we also saw how the "Living Water" was vitally important to our well-being. The same is true of light, when we talked about truth during our third study. Movement and walking with God came next. Now we're addressing the parallels between physical food and the "Bread of Life" that's freely offered by our loving Savior.

Notice that, when it comes to health, the physical laws set up at Creation are important enough. But those amazing spiritual implications—worship and relationship—are just as important—sometimes even more so! This will all come together for us as we move forward.

This week we're learning about God's original nutrition plan and why the world is so sick. We've also uncovered evidence from the likes of T. Colin Campbell and Caldwell Esselstyn that has revolutionized the medical world. And don't forget Daniel from the Old Testament and his story of eating healthy food when he was offered the best an entire nation had to offer. He knew even then that the wrong foods could be toxic and create stress in the body. He wanted no part of it!

Today, I want to focus on some texts highlighting food, specifically bread. Read these examples and circle the word "Bread" in each.

> But he answered, "It is written, 'Man shall not live by bread alone, but by every word that comes from the mouth of God. (Matthew 4:4)'
>
> Give us this day our daily bread. (Matthew 6:11; part of the Lord's Prayer)
>
> I am the bread of life. (John 6:48)
>
> Jesus then said to them, "Truly, truly, I say to you, it was not Moses who gave you the bread from heaven, but my Father gives you the true bread from heaven. For the bread of God is he who comes down from heaven and gives life to the world. (John 6:32,33)"

Yes, Jesus is the "Bread of Life." He became truth in human form. He understood that good nutrition is very important to the human body. And He taught nourishment comes from more than physical food. Look around you. We can clearly see the results of what occurs when the world strays from eating a plant-based diet. But we can also clearly see the results of not having Jesus, the Bread of Life, in hearts and minds. Look at the evidence. Look at the pain and suffering. Look at the sadness.

My journey as a cardiologist has gone through several stages. First, I simply wanted to get through school so I could save lives! I remember the long, long hours of studying and being at the hospital. I discovered I really loved doing procedures, making life and death decisions, and dealing with acute problems. I was completely focused on the physical issues of human existence.

As I matured and God worked in me, I began to realize that there was so much more I needed to know; more I needed to offer. In time, I turned to helping my patients make the very lifestyle changes that we've been studying in these lessons. I learned about nutrition and the brain. The more I learned, the more I needed to learn. I realized how beautiful and complex the human body is. The brain is such an important part of that puzzle yet so little is known about it.

Next, I studied Scripture, quickly realizing that technology will never be able to explain these complexities. Yes, we've sequenced the human genome. Yes, we've made brain-imaging possible. Yes, we know the chemical mechanisms of how plants change our physiology. But knowing is one thing. *Doing* is quite another. I needed my patients to start doing what I knew they needed to do.

God has also placed in us—in our fabric, in our DNA—a need to enjoy a relationship with our Creator. We can ignore it, cover it up with fast living, or douse it with strong doses of denial, but it's still there. When we finally give in and open our hearts to God, we still can't explain all the physiologic benefits from doing so. We just know that they happen. Accepting and believing in Jesus changes us from the inside out. But, do we have to know how or why? Not me. I'm just so glad it happens.

When we alter our diet, we can feel the changes taking place. When we invite Jesus into our hearts, the same thing happens. No explanation needed. Just praise.

Let's see if we can recognize some of the parallels between physical bread and inviting the Bread of Life into our lives. I'll present some aspects of physical bread and you write down what you think might be good examples of the same type of thing necessary for your spiritual life.

Physical Bread	Bread of Life
Your body needs nourishment	_____
You need to gather the ingredients	_____
It takes time to bake bread	_____
One wrong ingredient can spoil the loaf	_____
Baking requires heat	_____
Bread needs to be carefully preserved	_____
Bread can be easily shared with others	_____
When you eat bread, you can get full	_____
After eating bread, you'll get hungry in time	_____
Bread accepts many toppings	_____
Bread is best fresh from the oven	_____

I'd like to add something to this discussion about the parallels between physical bread and the Bread of Life. I've noticed something interesting about physical bread. It's not always the same and can look and taste very different in different parts of the world. There are the neatly sliced loaves found on most American super market shelves, the long, crusty loaves common in European countries, and the flat, round versions adorning tables in the Middle East. There's "sweet," "sour," "whole-grain," "French," and even "banana." Each shape and each type offers its own unique taste and texture. But they're all bread. They're all made with the same basic ingredients (flour, water, salt, and some type of leavening agent). It would be silly for me to say, "American bread is the *only* bread."

Sometimes, we try to wedge Christ—the Bread of Life—into a single category or shape or texture. "My personal understanding of God is the only God," we announce. But don't you think that the God of the universe is totally capable of making Himself accessible to and meeting the needs of *all* His children in *all* parts of the world? Sure, His health laws remain the same. If an Asian breaks one of those laws, the consequences are exactly the same as if a Canadian broke that law. And if a Russian refuses to enter into a relationship with the Creator, the end result exactly mirrors what would happen if an Argentinean did the same. So there are some "ingredients" of the Bread of Life that remain identical anywhere. But the way God looks—His "texture" and "taste"—can vary greatly. The Bible brings this fact out in clear detail. When His rebellious children needed an authoritative God, they got one. When we needed a sinless, spotless lamb to be offered on their behalf, Jesus became that for us., they got one. Sometimes He displays Himself as a Judge; sometimes as a forgiving Father; sometimes a tender husband. Same God, different textures.

My point is that, as we move along our journey to health—as we get to know the Bread of Life—we need to be open to the fact that some of our friends and family won't see things as we do. Some needs won't be the same as ours. That's why I like to stick with the basics. Fresh air, sunshine, movement, worship, nutrition, light—these needs, these "laws of health," don't change. But *how* people integrate these into their lives is up to them. I just share what I know in love, and let them bring these truths into their lives in ways—and in the time—they see fit. I invite you to do the same.

WRAPPING IT UP

Good nutrition, as we've been learning, is extremely valuable. The "Bread of Life"—Jesus—is priceless. Words cannot explain the worth. Technology is just beginning to offer insights into exactly what He has and is doing for us. We were designed by God and *for* God. He is our Ultimate Prescription.

LIVING IN COMMUNITY

We discussed in today's lesson the condition of the world. Write down and share your perception of how the world is doing today. Are Jesus and the Word being touted as the solution? Take some time and read the story of Noah. Are there parallels to our current situation?

BEING MISSIONAL

We learned that we need more than physical food. Sometimes, when we're sharing our witness, we experience a loss for words. That's OK, because words simply can't express how much God loves us.

I encourage you to follow in Christ's footsteps today and find an opportunity for the ministry of presence. Just be there for someone. Let them know you're praying for them. See if your group can find an opportunity to leave a Bible with someone who might need some spiritual bread.

COMMITMENT

Spend a few moments thanking and praising God for giving us truth and the ability to be healed. Write down your thanks and praises to God here:

_____

_____

Don't forget the other steps for good nutrition. Put a checkmark beside the ones you'll be incorporating this week:

- ❑ Drinking more water.

- ❑ Eating a bigger, healthier breakfast.

- ❑ Eating earlier and less at night.

- ❑ Enjoying 3-5 fruits and veggies each day.

- ❑ Making healthy snacks to carry with you.

- ❑ Being thankful for all of God's blessings.

DAY 6

What was Wrong with Manna?

I hope you had a good night's rest. This week is flying by as we've been studying nutrition together. It only makes sense that we learn about building and maintaining optimum health from our Creator. He should know exactly what's best for us. That's why He did what He did during those amazing days of Creation Week. That story never gets old to me; because it's here that we find the health laws that govern our very existence. It's here that we discover the cures for so many of our ills. Thank you God for including details of that incredible week in your Holy Word.

As you remember from reading the Old Testament, when the Israelites left Egypt, they needed a food source and they needed it *now*! A plant-based diet was not available. After all, they were out in the middle of a very arid, unforgiving desert. So, what did God do? He supplied them with an alternative crop called "manna." As a matter of fact, God fed His people for forty years with this heaven-sent food. Let's examine the account found in the book of Exodus.

In the first verse of Exodus chapter 16, the liberated Israelites started to grumble—and for good reason. They were hungry. It's pretty hard to remain civil when you're hungry. Anyone with children knows that to be true. But, I'll have to say that it's hard for me to fathom how the Israelites, who'd just witnessed great miracles such as the parting of the Red Sea, could be found grumbling and not trusting God. But, that was the case. Let's start reading in verse four:

> Then the Lord said to Moses, "Behold, I am about to rain bread from heaven for you, and the people shall go out and gather a day's portion every day, that I may test them, whether they will walk in my law or not. On the sixth day, when they prepare what they bring in, it will be twice as much as they gather daily." So Moses and Aaron said to all the people of Israel, "At evening you shall know that it was the Lord who brought you out of the land of Egypt, and in the morning you shall see the glory of the Lord, because he has heard your grumbling against the Lord. For what are we, that you grumble against us? (Exodus 16:4-7)"

In other words, "Hey, don't shoot the messenger!" Let's continue:

> When the people of Israel saw it, they said to one another, "What is it?" For they did not know what it was. And Moses said to them, "It is the bread that the Lord has given you to eat. This is what the Lord has commanded: 'Gather of it, each one of you, as much as he can eat. You shall each take an omer, according to the number of the persons that each of you has in his tent. (Exodus 16:15,16)"

An "omer" is about 123 ounces (3.64 liters).

As the chapter continues God gave specific instructions concerning how and when to gather the manna. He told them to gather enough for their household until the sixth day and, in preparation for the coming Sabbath, they were to gather twice as much. If they gathered twice as much on the other days, it would spoil. Obedience was and still is important to God.

> Now the house of Israel called its name manna. It was like coriander seed, white, and the taste of it was like wafers made with honey. Moses said, "This is what the Lord has commanded: 'Let an omer of it be kept throughout your generations, so that they may see the bread with which I fed you in the wilderness, when I brought you out of the land of Egypt. (Exodus 16:31,32)"

God supplied their nutritional needs with manna. He also wanted their obedience and for them to remember in the future how He provided food for them in the middle of a dry, dangerous desert. They ate this miraculous food for forty years. And guess what? There were no reports of nutritionally related problems.

Manna was like dew; it melted in the sun. I'd love to know the nutrient composition of this amazing source of sustenance. But I can guarantee you that there were no chemicals or preservatives hidden inside. Also, notice God gave them something that was fresh each and every day.

But, as is often the case in the human condition, the Israelites couldn't just be thankful and move on. No, they had to grumble and complain as they journeyed down the dusty road toward the Promised Land.

> Now the rabble that was among them had a strong craving. And the people of Israel also wept again and said, "Oh that we had meat to eat! We remember the fish we ate in Egypt that cost nothing, the cucumbers, the melons, the leeks, the onions, and the garlic. But now our strength is dried up, and there is nothing at all but this manna to look at." Now the manna was like coriander seed, and its appearance like that of bdellium. (Numbers 11:4-7)

"Bdellium" is a semi-transparent resin. Notice that the "mixed multitude" (those of different ancestry that escaped out of Egypt with them) started the complaining and the Israelites joined in. Moses was feeling the pressure and in verse 14 stated that he couldn't bear it alone. Evidently this feeling for some flesh foods was intense. In verse 18, the Lord gave in to their complaining and provided meat to eat: quail. The result for those who craved and ate the meat wasn't so good. It reports in verse 33 that a very great plague struck. Sound familiar? When we move away from God's original prescriptions for life, there's a price to pay—not because God is punishing us, but because we aren't giving our bodies what they need to survive and thrive.

What can we learn from this story? I believe there are several take-home messages:

- Good nutrition is a gift from God.

- Even in the wilderness He will supply our needs.

- Don't cave-in to those around us who might start the grumbling.

- Obedience is important to God.

- We might, at times, not understand why God is asking us to live a certain way, to go on a certain path, or read and apply a particular scripture. But we can rest assured that it is in our best interest because God is motivated by love and cares a great deal for His wayward children. Those with children can certainly understand that our kids often do not understand or heed our advice, but we give direction because we love them.

WRAPPING IT UP

God gives nutritional recommendations because He loves us. It might not be wise to cave-in to advertisements, commercials, and cultural influences even though, in the short term, that seems to be the easiest path to take. I try to keep in mind that advertisers aren't concerned with my health. They're concerned with their bottom line and are perfectly willing to sacrifice me in order to make a profit.

Think about and discus some of the commercials you've seen on television or online. What four main benefits do they seem to promise you if you'll just use their products:

1. _____

2. _____

3. _____

4. _____

In what ways does God provide the very same benefits, but through building good health and happiness?"

1. _____

2. _____

3. _____

4. _____

LIVING IN COMMUNITY

The Israelites lived in a large community. Think about and discuss four of the main issues they might have faced living in a wilderness.

1. _____
2. _____
3. _____
4. _____

- Do we have these same issues today?

- In what ways are we in a "wilderness" waiting to cross into the Promised Land?

Knowing the needs of community in general, make a short list of some of the physical and spiritual "manna" we can provide as we attempt to be an encourager to our group—and beyond.

_____
_____
_____
_____

Also, don't forget to share with the group a recipe, restaurant, store or ideas that can help improve everyone's nutrition.

BEING MISSIONAL

What was the biggest take-home point for you in the lesson? To me, it was that manna was more than food. It was a chance to be obedient and follow the instructions of our Heavenly Father. As you interact with those in your group, family or neighborhood today, keep in mind that your manna could offer multiple benefits. Also, pray that we all can reach the Promised Land soon.

COMMITMENT

Poor Moses. He had to put up with so much! I hope I never burden those around me with complaining. Next time you want to complain, do what I try to do. Find two things to praise God about and then thank Him for the bread of life provided new each and every day.

We're nearing the end of the week. How is your food chart coming along? Being aware of what's being included is so important. Have you made some simple changes? Are you committed to learning more? In one short week, we can only touch the surface. I hope you'll continue to search for evidence and information that will make your journey all the good things it can be.

As we've seen, there are spiritual blessings in following God's plan for nutrition.

DAY 7

Your Day of Rest

Rest is a gift. It's the very opposite of stress. Rest produces changes and chemicals we can now quantitate.

There's **physical** rest:

• Resting at night and letting our individual cells recover from doing their jobs.

• Resting our muscles with a walk in the woods or nap on the couch.

• Resting our gastro-intestinal system by actually stopping eating.

• Resting our eyes and ears by switching off the computer or television set.

We were designed to have down time. Without physical rest, stress chemistry takes over.

There's **mental** rest:

• Allowing the brain some down time by ceasing work and worry.

• Stopping feeding the brain information that it needs to remember.

• Spending time in God's Word instead of facing a constant media barrage.

• Imaging peaceful scenes in our thoughts instead of replaying disappointments.

There's **spiritual** rest:

• Communing with the Creator.

• Worshiping at church or in nature.

• Listening to uplifting Christian music.

• Spending time in quiet reflection and prayer.

All of these types of rests offer endless physiologic benefits. Next week, we'll dive into the brain and the incredible blessings of worship.

Summary of week 5

1. God's nutritional recommendations at Creation are still relevant.

2. Evidence-based studies support God's Biblical RX for nutrition.

3. There are blessings in following God's plan.

4. Our nutrition is medicinal.

5. Nutrition for the soul is more than the food we eat.

6. God's gifts are good even if we don't understand them. A little faith goes a long way.

7.   Rest is vital. We ignore it at our own peril..

Today, make the time to rest physically, mentally, and spiritually. God bless.

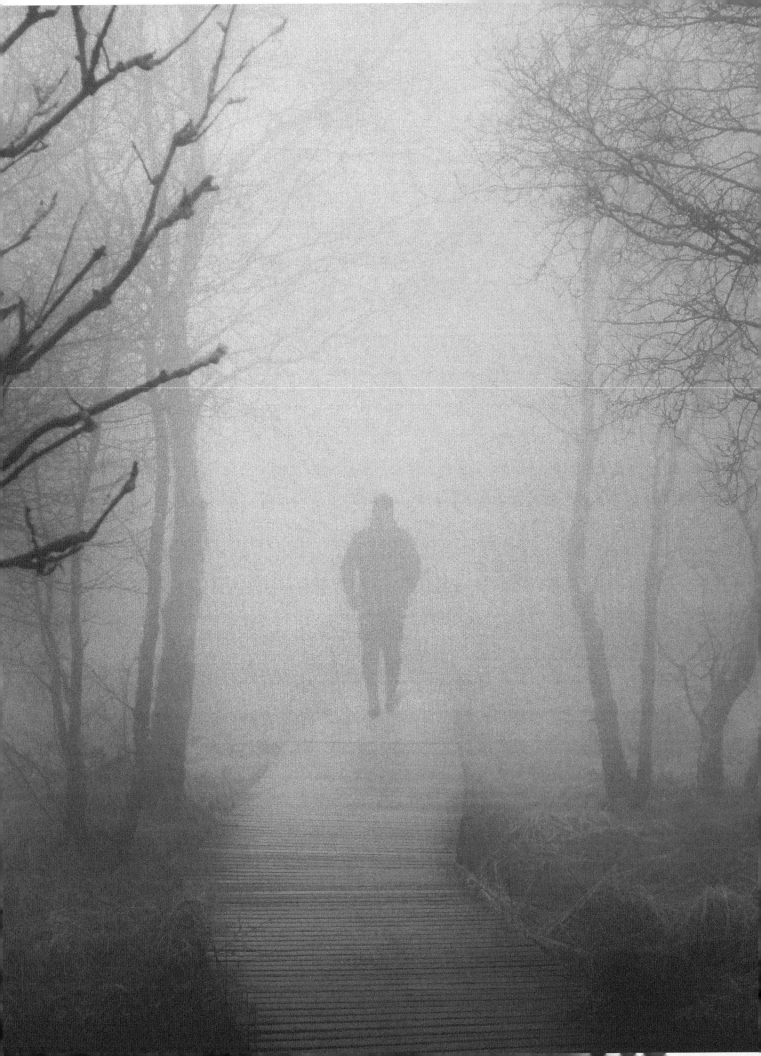

WEEK 6

Biblical Prescriptions for Life 5—Healing Begins in Our Heads

Jane was distraught. Actually, distraught was an understatement. She was more like crushed, ashamed, hurt, depressed, confused, angry, and stressed. She couldn't escape her feelings—and for a pretty good reason. She'd found her husband of eleven years with another woman. Not only was she working a forty-hour week, she was taking care of three young children on top of all that.

She and her husband had not communicated well for a quite a while, leaving her frightened for the future. All of these emotions were causing her brain to be overloaded with fear and anxiety.

When she asked for advice, I believed the greatest value I could provide her was to simply listen, using the ministry of presence. Where do you start when your world is upside down, your brain is on overload, and you can't concentrate, eat, do a good job at work or raise children? Some of you reading this may have had a similar experience.

These situations are so complicated, and yet, this is life!

As we've been studying together these weeks, I hope the first place we've learned to turn for help—for clarity, for hope, for some sense of normalcy—Great Physician. "God is our refuge and strength, a very present help in trouble" (Psalm 46.1). Notice, this truth is a promise from God that He will be present with us in whatever difficulties come our way. We can trust Him. I asked Jane if she'd done this. She responded that she had turned to God, but wasn't hearing His voice or feeling His comfort.

I began to talk to her about what her brain was going through. The tremendous stress had activated the amygdala as well as limbic system where emotions are generated. Alarms were sounding. The amygdala was doing its job, preparing the body to survive. The "fight or flight" response was in full readiness. The brain just wanted to survive. This response was programmed into Jane's DNA.

This constant chemical bombardment was not helping her situation. The adrenaline, cortisol, cytokines, and inflammatory proteins were speeding up her heart, raising her blood pressure, causing her to lose sleep. Her appetite was gone and her body ached. But, the most significant problem was that she could not think rationally. When we're angry and under stress, our cognitive abilities are diminished. When stress chemistry is dominating, the brain simply wants to be safe, to stay alive. The higher functioning parts of the brain in the pre-frontal cortex are blunted as the body fights for survival.

Can you remember your mom instructing you to take a few deep breaths and relax when you were angry? Well, she was right! There are chemical changes that take place just from taking a few deep breaths helping us to relax.

I explained to Jane that God was there ready to help, but to even recognize His presence, she needed to utilize more of her pre-frontal cortex and less of her amygdala. How could she do that? This week we'll be learning and studying about the brain, how it works, and how God can "create in us a new mind." We will discover what we can do when our lives are so disturbed that the brain is "out of whack." What do we do when the organ we need most is being damaged by stress? We will also learn that there is a real battle for the control of our brain and this battle is constantly raging.

Thus far in our lessons, we've implemented many Biblical Prescriptions that help the brain function better, enabling a better connection with God. Whether this is through water, light, movement, or good nutrition, each is effective and necessary. But what happens when our world is crumbling from a broken relationship, an illness, a death, loss of a job, or a shaken belief system? What do we need to do when we are so "shaken" that the part of the brain we need most is not functioning at an optimal level?

What are some practical steps we can take if and when this happens to us? Hopefully, by the end of the week, we'll have a prescription, a strategy, a plan, a software program uploaded to help us—and those we hold dear. What are the brain skills we need to enhance? How do we recognize the battle for our brains? What are the needed Biblical Prescriptions?

We have much to cover. Review the video again. I will be reinforcing those points during the week. The brain is complicated, but by learning about our "control center," we'll be ready to face the uncertainties of life just a little better. Let's stop for a moment to thank and praise God, asking Him for help and clarity as we learn and study together.

God, there are many in this world who, like Jane, have what seems to be insurmountable problems. Some in this very place might have this stress. As we come to You, we pray that You will open our eyes to truth. We know You are with us. As we grow in You, teach us what to do when our lives are turned upside down. Amen.

VIDEO GUIDE 6

Healing from the Top Down

VIDEO (20 minutes)

Major Bible verses:

- Philippians 4:6

- Romans 12

- 2 Corinthians 10:5

- Romans 8

Who is Jane? _____

What stands out to you about her? _____

Is there anything in her life you can relate to?:

Age _____

Symptoms_____

Lifestyle_____

Relationships_____

Where do many symptoms originate? _____

Does science support this? _____

What Jane experienced	What it meant
• quickened heart rate	_____
• shallow breathing	_____
• perspiration	_____
• jumbled thoughts	_____

Does stress in the mind stay in the mind?_____

Is it possible for the brain to stressed to the point of shutdown? _____

The brain can be divided into the Upper Brain, Middle Brain and Lower Brain. Generally speaking, what are the processes associated with each division?

Division	Processes
• Lower Brain	_____
• Middle Brain	_____
• Upper Brain	_____

Sometimes one part of the brain is used more than another part. This has been described by brain experts as "downshifting" or "upshifting" to a different gear.

What are the characteristics of this process?

Downshift Mode   **Upshift Mode**

_____   _____
_____   _____
_____   _____
_____   _____
_____   _____

Can you describe a time when you've experienced downshifting? _____

Are there specific triggers which cause you to downshift? Be specific:

_____

_____

_____

_____

Just as Jane demonstrated how our minds could negatively impact our physiology, we've learned that it's possible to improve our body's chemistry by upshifting to a higher division of the brain. When we purposefully upshift, we change the immediate state of our body and mind. As we practice the discipline of upshifting, over time God can actually re-wire our neural pathways, releasing us from repetitive, destructive thoughts and habits. A large component of health is "in the mind." In this lesson, we'll discover a process by which neural pathways are established and reinforced.

Biblical Prescriptions for Life for Week 6

1. _____

2. _____

3. _____

4. _____

Group Discussion (20 Minutes)

• What most impacted you most during the video? Why? _____

• Describe the way you feel when you are downshifted. _____

• How often do you think you are downshifted in the course of a regular day? _____

• Are you down shifted right now? _____

• What are the triggers that cause you to downshift? _____

- When do you find yourself downshifted? Do you recognize what is happening to you?

  _____

- In what situations do you believe you have the choice between upshifting and downshifting? _____

  _____

- If you chose to stay downshifted, what kinds of thoughts are you focused upon?

  _____

And now, with your group, finish this sentence—"*I want to change* _____"

LIVING IN COMMUNITY

We've saved some of the most profound Biblical Prescriptions for Life for week six. That's partly because it takes time to change—one step, then two, then three. As we change, we're empowered to continue the journey. God empowers us through a relationship with Him. These changes may help lower blood pressure and heart rate, decrease risk of infection, help with blood sugar or sleep problems; the list goes on. Biblical Prescriptions change the chemistry of the entire body.

For this reason, students are experiencing meaningful changes as they continue *Biblical Prescriptions for Life*. I hope you're also growing together in your relationships as your bodies grow healthier.

Take time in your small group to ask your study buddy and other members how you can serve them this week as they integrate this Biblical Prescription for Life.

Name	The Best Way I Can Care for Them	Mobile Number

INDIVIDUAL REFLECTION

As we listen to each other, what is your top-level take away from this weeks' time together? This is just for you. Write it here. _____

BEING MISSIONAL

Listen to the way people speak to themselves and others this week. Pray for the right opportunity to be loving, encouraging, and hopeful to those around you. The real, persistent change in your life will open the door to supernatural conversations—when the time is right. Remember, *Biblical Prescriptions for Life* is a way to healing and wellness. None of us have arrived. Remain humble and gracious. Perhaps you can start a *Biblical Prescriptions for Life* study group with people from your office or school. "God has not given us a Spirit of Fear" (2 Timothy 1:7).

COMMITMENT

"This week, I am going to ADD and DO at least one of the following simple Biblical Prescriptions for Life:"

I commit to	Biblical Prescriptions for Life	Day 1	2	3	4	5	6	7
	Read aloud 5x each day. Practice, memorize & recite:							
	Philippians 4:8 *"Finally, brothers, whatsoever is true, whatever is honorable, whatever is just, whatever is pure, whatever is lovely, whatever is commendable, if there is ant excellence, if there is anything worthy of praise, think about these things."*							
	Romans 8:5-6 *"For those who live according to the flesh set their minds to the things of the flesh, but those who live according to the Spirit set their minds on the things of the Spirit. For to set the mind on the flesh is death, but to set the mind on the Spirit is life and peace."*							
	Journal My Thoughts each day this week							
	Downshifted thinking focused on:							
	Downshifted thinking triggered by:							
	Downshifted thinking perpetuated by:							
	I chose to upshift my thinking about _____ by:							
	I chose to retrain my neural pathway on this (person/subject/ situation _____) by replacing it with this truth _____.							

If you missed a session or want to review one, go to biblicalprescriptionsforlife.com to stream Dr. Marcum's audio and video.

DAY 1

Be Anxious For Nothing

God, through Philippians 4:6, admonishes us to be anxious about nothing. In examining Jane's situation, she was definitely anxious. God knows that anxiety was not good for the brain. Think back to the last time you were anxious. How did you feel? What did you do?

Before we move on, I think we need to understand exactly what anxiety is. Anxiety is a word. But, what does this word represent? Mere words can't really explain what's going on inside of us as we deal with the complexities of life. How does this emotion change our brain? How do we even explain an emotion? Why is anxiety dangerous to our health? God knew this was going to be a problem and He gave a Biblical Prescription.

Anxiety is a form of fear. Fear is one of the four core emotions: fear, anger, joy, and sadness. We use the word "emotion" to try to explain the chemistry that the body produces in response to various stimuli. The words we use to try to explain emotions are inadequate to capture the true physiology. In the case of Jane, she might have had 70% fear, 20% anger and 10% sadness. I doubt she had any joy. I hope I haven't made this too complicated, but the brain is a complicated organ. However, the more we can learn, the more we'll understand how God can, not only heal a brain, but create a new one in us!

Anxiety is an emotion that can occur when the brain feels threatened. It's a very common emotion and runs a spectrum from a little anxious to *a lot* of anxious. The brain processes the experience we're facing and determines the overall threat. What happens next is vitally important.

Before I go on, let me give you a little peek into the complexity of the brain. This will help you understand that we mere mortals really know very little about the brain. When God instructs us to be "anxious about nothing" and to "not have a spirit of fear," how do we do that when our brain is screaming: "Be anxious, be afraid!"

The brain is the most complex three-pound object in the solar system. It consists of 100 billion neurons with a quadrillion (that's 1 with 15 zeros after it) interconnections. These neurons and interconnections are constantly processing information, downloading memories from the hippocampus and constantly evaluating the environment while trying to maintain life. Twenty three thousand genes control the neurons and connections. Just a few genes seem to drive intelligence. Our genome—twenty-three thousand genes—seems much too small for the job.

Egyptians thought the brain was a useless organ. Aristotle thought the soul was in the heart. But, now we understand that when the Bible mentions the heart, it's really referring to the brain or the mind—the center of our thinking, feeling, choosing and reasoning.

The brain uses 20% of our total energy, sometimes less, sometimes more. Sixty-five percent of the energy expenditure within a newborn is for brain function. More has been learned about the brain in the last 15 years than in the history of the planet. I could go on, but I think you get the picture.

Stress accelerates the death of new neurons and changes the way the brain functions. Anxiety and fear are stressors and actually change the physical and chemical structures of the brain. Stress also shifts the priorities, sometimes downshifting to the lower, stay alive, be selfish, live in the present, part of the brain. This was what was happening to Jane in our story.

Fear, cowardice, anxiety, apprehension, agitation, dread, fretting, fright, worry, uneasiness, troubled, distressed, angst, uneasiness, strained, nervousness, are all words used to try to explain how the brain processes our environment.

There are many types of anxiety and phobias.

- Fear of crowds (denophobia)
- Fear of beards (pogonophobia)
- Fear of people (anthophobia)
- Fear of the sun (heliophobia)
- Fear of God (theophobia)
- Fear of snow (chionophobia)
- Fear of dirt (mysophobia)

The list goes on and on. Paranoia is ramped up anxiety. Obsessive-compulsive disorder and panic attacks are forms of anxiety. Then, there is the severest form: post-traumatic stress. All are forms of fear and put stress on our system.

It's estimated that one in three people will, in a lifetime, experience some form of anxiety and 17% have anxiety at any one time. As I explained earlier, stress and anxiety damage the brain, especially over the long haul. The extent to which anxiety and fear—even of the unknown—can damage health should not be underestimated.

A true study has been told of a patient with a liver mass who believed that the mass was a malignancy. The physicians didn't want to perform a biopsy as the lesion was small and in a difficult location. So, they recommended observation of the lesion with serial scans. The patient feared cancer and was constantly pressing for other opinions. The lesion, which was discovered incidentally, dominated his thoughts. That belief or fear of a perceived danger brought consequences. He died in a year, and at the autopsy, they examined the lesion. It was benign. The patient had no pathology that should have caused his demise.

Then, there are the Pacific Islanders who die at the hand of witch doctors. They, too, die with no identifiable adverse pathology. Yes, the brain has a powerful effect on the body and Jane was under such extreme stress that her pre-frontal cortex was not working well. This was hindering her ability to connect with God

Remember:

- Fear and anxiety were not part of our original design.
- Stress chemistry downshifts our brain to the "let's stay alive" functions.
- The brain wants to feel safe.
- The cognitive part of the brain is under-utilized during stress.
- The physical and chemical changes generated by anxiety cause inflammation, genetic alterations, and activation—to some degree—of the "fight or flight" chemistry.

Extreme stress can stimulate so much epinephrine that heart attacks are induced. This is usually the stress generated by the loss of a loved one and is called the "Broken Heart Syndrome." Needless to say, mental stress affects the entire body.

WRAPPING IT UP

In the world today, fear abounds. Every input into our body has a chemical consequence. consequence. When we choose to be "anxious about nothing," when we refuse to be fearful, we're moving toward the spirit that God wants us to have. We were created to depend on and trust God for all of our needs. This moves us toward the prefrontal cortex, the part of the brain where God communicates with us.

This week we will also be developing strategies to upload so we can avoid the dangerous chemistry of fear.

LIVING IN COMMUNITY

Reach out to your study buddy today and ask how they see the anxiety and fear in their life. Maybe you can share an experience when you were fearful, and how you dealt with that situation. Then take time to pray for each other.

This is going to be a transformational week of study!

BEING MISSIONAL

The mission field isn't necessarily "out there" somewhere. For many of us, the mission field begins in our living room or the cubicle next to ours. Pray for opportunities to share good news and Biblical truth as God teaches you this week. But only share when you're motivated by love and can do it with gentleness and humility. Otherwise, we can do more harm than good if others perceive arrogance, self-righteousness or judgment in our witness. Remember, we're all learning together.

COMMITMENT

Take a look at your Biblical Prescriptions for Life commitments from week one through this week. Are you continuing to practice the simple actions from the first five weeks as you move ahead? If not, don't be critical of yourself. As we'll learn this week—that will down shift your brain!

Instead, consider if you've tried to bring too much change into your life at one time. Or, it may be an issue of keeping your motivation by reminding yourself of your desire for healing and life-long wellness. If you want it, no matter what yesterday was like, you can start again today. Spend some tome today memorizing Philippians 4:6.

DAY 2

Strategies to Upshift Out of Anxiety and Fear

Today we're going to review some of the principles presented in the video. Then, we'll provide some strategies to help up-shift our brains. As we remember, our brains just want to be safe. This is an adaptive mechanism built into our DNA. We must survive. That's why our brains have mechanisms hard-wired for protection and safety.

In the late 1960's, Dr. Paul MacLean described three functional layers of the brain. This was remarkable in that he made this discovery before the development of brain imaging with CT scans, PET scans, EEG's, and functional MRI's. He was far ahead of his time. A quick review will be helpful before we learn some strategies for anxiety.

I had a roommate who once had a pet boa constrictor. He told me how much his snake loved him. I had to laugh, as reptiles live in the lower brain—the reptilian brain. They live entirely in the present. Their top concerns are safety, food, and reproducing. This part of the brain does have sensory layers for the reptile to monitor the environment, but they don't possess emotions, remember the past, or plan for the future. It is all about the "here and now."

This is the "me first," selfish part of the brain that we share with these creatures. When we're under extreme stress, our brains shift to this "stay-alive" section where the need for security and safety is paramount. It makes us want to run from danger. When this part is dominant, the stress chemicals epinephrine, cortisol, cytokines and other inflammatory mediators predominate. Under its influence, we really don't think or plan ahead.

Dr. MacLean calls the next layer "mammalian." This is the part of the brain that we share with mammals. My pet dogs, Max and Daphne, definitely have mammalian brains. This is where the sense of smell resides and my dogs are great at smelling things. This part of the brain also contains the limbic system where emotions reside. This layer is also very fast, and can actually illicit a response before the "thinking brain," the prefrontal cortex, has time to modulate the response. Many crimes of passion occur under the control of this layer. The "mammalian" brain also houses immune system responses. The hippocampus, the search engine part of the brain, where memories are stored, also reside within this layer. It's here that we recognize and remember the past.

Thanks to our mammalian layer, when an emotional situation develops, sometimes actions occur before the thinking part of the brain gets involved. This layer recognizes that other creatures exist, but still is not involved in future planning. My dogs never think ahead. They just love to smell, recognize me, and remember that I'm the one filling their bowls with food. Their wagging tails and licking tongues demonstrate their emotions. Just think. Emotions, memories, and immune system function reside in a brain layer void of conscious thought.

The third functional layer is the new brain, the neocortex or pre-frontal cortex. Some mammals have some neocortexes—dolphins, crows, and some primates—but this layer is mostly unique to humans. This part of the brain boasts the anterior cingulate cortex known as the "God brain." (More on that next week.)

This layer has a left and right side, is capable of abstract thought, empathetic deeds, plans ahead, loves, and is where our consciousness resides. It's great at problem solving, metaphors, and sophisticated thinking. This is also where we plan for the future. As we learn more about this part of the brain, we'll discover that it's here we should want to focus our energies the most. Why? Because this is the part of the brain that communicates with God. The steps we have taken the last few weeks has helped each one of us improve this part of the brain. Less stress in our life means we are improving the prefrontal cortex.

Studies have shown that when we are in crisis mode or totally stressed out, we retain less than 15% of what we're told. We lose the ability to discern cause and effect and problem solve. The stressed brain ages faster and all the stress chemicals increase the risk of heart attack, suppress the immune system, and reactivate old behaviors.

For example, when a person is stressed, what does he or she do to feel better? If working predominantly from the mammalian layer, out may come the pack of cigarettes, or the six-pack of beer, or enough donuts to supply a satisfying "pig out". However, if working from the third layer of the brain, that same person might think first and look for positive, less harmful ways to cope with the stress.

In Philippians 4:6, we read: "Be anxious for nothing, but in everything by prayer and supplication, with thanksgiving, let your requests be made known to God." This Biblical Prescription for Life upshifts our brains and results in much prayer and a coming to God for the needed answers.

When David was stressed to the max, he came to God and recognized he needed a new brain. Next week we will focus on the science of worship, but for today, as we think about what anxiety and fear does to our brains, let's look for some practical approaches.

First, evaluate the concern. Is the fear valid? Most episodes of anxiety occur when an individual overreacts to a situation, jumps to a conclusion without evaluating all the facts, or starts taking things personally. But, when those same fears are evaluated by the cognitive function of the brain, they're often seen as solvable, and not a problem at all. The stress chemistry is turned off. The threat wasn't really life threatening at all, hardly worth the time and effort spent thinking about it.

In Jane's case, here are the cognitive steps that I recommended:

1. **Pray** to God and ask for help.

2. **Worship** as outlined in next week's lesson.

3. **Remember** how God has cared for you in the past.

4. Learn to **breathe deeply.** Draw in a deep breath, hold for two seconds, and blow it out slowly. Do this for ten minutes. This activates the parasympathetic nervous system and turns down the stress chemistry.

5. Find three things to be **thankful** for.

6. Find two things to **laugh** about. Do a hippocampus search and reactivate a belly-laughing experience you enjoy remembering.

7. Check for **health factors** that may be contributing to your stress such as lack of water, movement, or sleep. A movement strategy might be needed. A toxin might be contributing.

As Jane developed her pre-planned strategy for stress, her brain rebooted and moved to the cognitive layer where she could focus on worship. She discovered that she could live in that part of her brain, her "new brain" that God created to communicate with us. She now had a software program to upload. Whenever she felt stress, the program could be loaded 1,2,3,4,5,6, and 7. She literally learned how to throw away stress!

Second Timothy 1:7 reads: "God has not given us a spirit of fear, but of power and of love and of a sound mind." This is what I see as a major problem in today's world. Fear abounds. Look at the evidence. We all need a sound mind; a brain not stressed out and functioning at the lower levels. We desire—and God desires for us—a brain functioning at a higher level, giving us power to make changes, learning to love and not be selfish, and overcoming the stresses of the world.

To change the way you feel, you must change your thoughts. Feelings follow thoughts. It takes around 7 seconds for a thought to get to your consciousness, where you actually know what your brain is thinking. Many thoughts are in your brain all the time. Most thoughts you never know about because they are not making it to your consciousness, yet they are inducing physiologic changes. You may have developed, over time, negative thinking styles. These negative thoughts may be bouncing around changing your physiology without your awareness. You might be living in a stressed out brain. The brain is complex.

I think when you find your brain stressed, the simple steps outlined above is a great place to start. These steps will allow you to move on instead of hanging on. Today is the day to learn and change. I want to close our lesson by having you say out loud, I John 4:18: "Love casts out all fear."

Love originates in that higher functioning layer. You grow in knowing God through worshipping Him, just as you are doing right now. But, be warned, there is a battle for control of our brain and tomorrow we will study more about this.

WRAPPING IT UP

If you are stressed, remember our lesson today.

How has this lesson affected you? Are you empowered, enlightened, hopeful, or encouraged? We covered a lot of ground. In a single day, we tried to gain a new perspective on a complicated subject. Yes, we're made in God's image—that includes having a spiritual nature—we're designed to have a relationship with our Creator. The answer to fear is found in this relationship.

Write down your take-home points from today's lesson.

_____

_____

_____

LIVING IN COMMUNITY

Our spiritual perceptions can get challenged each and every day. The physical world "feels" more real. The physical world's demands seem more critical. The risk and reward system in the material world seems more immediate and tangible. But, all of this can distract us from the bigger story.

Today, make a point to call your study buddy and perhaps a few others from your study group to encourage them to look with "spiritual eyes" for the big picture in the here and now. Remind them that we can help each other. Remind them that God the Father guarantees that He will create in us a new mind.

Based on this lesson, what changes can you make today when you feel anxious?

_____

How have you been handling fear and anxiety in your life?

_____

BEING MISSIONAL

This week, a big part of being missional is keeping your personal focus on the larger spiritual reality. Spend quality time talking to God about your doubts and fears. Spend quality time re-reading the Bible passages from this week's study. Be ready to strengthen your small group with God's word. Be positive.

COMMITMENT

The writer of Psalms (literally, "songs") knew the importance of memorizing God's word in the battle for their heart and mind. Listen to what he wrote in Psalm 119:9-16:

> How can a young man keep his way pure?
>> By guarding it according to your word.
>
> With my whole heart I seek you;
>> let me not wander from your commandments!
>
> I have stored up your word in my heart,
>> that I might not sin against you.
>
> Blessed are you, O Lord;
>> teach me your statutes!
>
> With my lips I declare
>> all the rules of your mouth.
>
> In the way of your testimonies I delight
>> as much as in all riches.

I will meditate on your precepts
    and fix my eyes on your ways.

I will delight in your statutes;
    I will not forget your word.

I encourage you to work on your memorization to charge your truth battery. Keep journaling your thoughts to get a picture of the very real battle for your heart and mind.

DAY 3

The Ultimate War

We started this week by expanding our knowledge of how the brain works. Proper mental function is vital to our physical health. Today, we're going to look at some big-picture concepts. God wants us to be "anxious about nothing" and to turn our minds to Him. We're learning how to do this. However, there's another force wanting to control our minds, to create stress, to go against our very design. This force causes physical problems—both in the short and long term.

In 2003, the world was a very different place from the one in which I grew up. We were two years past the 9/11 terrorist attacks that rocked the American sense of domestic security. There was a new type of war—The War on Terror—that transcended geography, economy, education and politics. Alexander T.J. Lennon coined the phrase, "the battle for hearts and minds" when he wrote about using soft power (i.e., influence, benevolence, community building instead of firepower, sanctions and intimidation) to win this type of war.

Although it's too early to understand how history will judge our motives and actions in the post-9/11 world, Lennon was onto a very significant set of much larger truths. The Bible identifies a war that's being fought in the realm of ideas and "powers and principalities" (Ephesians 6). And the battleground—the territory under dispute— is in our hearts and minds. As we study this week, let's remember the steps we need to take when our brains are being threatened. The same steps we take to combat fear can be applied to the battle—the *spiritual* war—that goes on each day of our life. Hopefully we're aware of the war. That awareness is the big picture item I want to stress today.

This pivotal truth—that there is a war going on for our brains—finds its foundation in the very words of God (see below). You see, God cares about our *heart* (the brain—the center of our emotions, thoughts and desires). This is the very place where He communicates with us. Our actions and our chemistry originate in the brain. In fact, it's our mind that reveals who we really are and who or what we truly worship. As we've been learning, our physical health and brain health are interconnected.

So, what does Scripture say about the mind? Deuteronomy 6:4, 5 reads: "Hear, O Israel: The Lord our God, the Lord is one. You shall love the Lord your God with all your heart and with all your soul and with all your might."

This brings us to the importance of treating the mind and understanding the inputs influencing our thoughts. Today, I want to make sure we comprehend the big picture of the war: who the enemy is, the weapons he uses, the theatre in which the battles rage and the goals he has set.

As we study God's Word, it all becomes crystal clear. This war is as real—if not more real—than any conflict we'll see in the news. There's even an explanation for *why* we don't see this war in the nightly news.

First, it's very important that we acknowledge that the spiritual battle is not evident to many people. In fact, most will reject the idea outright. We need supernatural perception to get a grasp of this reality. Listen to what the Apostle Paul wrote to one of the churches he founded. They too were grappling with big issues that went beyond the empirical world.

> The natural person does not accept the things of the Spirit of God, for they are folly to him, and he is not able to understand them because they are spiritually discerned. The spiritual person judges all things, but is he to be judged by no one. "For who has understood the mind of the Lord so as to instruct him?" But we have the mind of Christ. (1 Corinthians 2:14-16)

Second, our enemy doesn't want us to know we're at war. That's because people who don't believe they're at war don't live with a mental readiness or a vigilance. They get mentally and physically soft. Others do the thinking for them. As you remember day one and two of this week, we were designed to worship the true God. However, *other* worship can take control of our brain causing stress and "bad chemistry." This masks reality.

For these two reasons, we need spiritual understanding. Let's pause for prayer.

> *Father, since the dawn of time You have suffered rebellion against your loving, right rule. There has been a struggle between those who trust you as God and those who want to be god. Adam and Eve chose to go their own way—Eve was deceived and Adam chose rebellion. Since that time, there's been a war between those two kingdoms. Help us begin to understand the reality we can't see with our eyes, and accept how this unseen reality affects our very health. We pray for wisdom and strength to follow and worship You. Amen.*

Read the following passages and then answer the questions that follow

> Finally, be strong in the Lord and in the strength of his might. Put on the whole armor of God, that you may be able to stand against the schemes of the devil. For we do not wrestle against flesh and blood, but against the rulers, against the authorities, against the cosmic powers over this present darkness, against the spiritual forces of evil in the heavenly places. (Ephesians 6:10-12)

> Humble yourselves, therefore, under the mighty hand of God so that at the proper time He may exalt you, casting all your anxieties on Him, because He cares for you. Be sober-minded; be watchful. Your adversary the devil

prowls around like a roaring lion, seeking someone to devour. Resist him, firm in your faith, knowing that the same kinds of suffering are being experienced by your brotherhood throughout the world. (1 Peter 5:6-9)

Who is our Enemy? _____

Is there more than one? _____

How would you recognize them?_____

What are the resources and weapons our enemy uses to control our mind? _____

But I say, walk by the Spirit, and you will not gratify the desires of the flesh. For the desires of the flesh are against the Spirit, and the desires of the Spirit are against the flesh, for these are opposed to each other, to keep you from doing the things you want to do. (Galatians 5:16, 17)

What causes quarrels and what causes fights among you? Is it not this that your passions are at war within you? You desire and do not have, so you murder. You covet and cannot obtain, so you fight and quarrel. You do not have, because you do not ask. You ask and do not receive, because you ask wrongly, to spend it on your passions. You adulterous people! Do you not know that friendship with the world is enmity with God? Therefore whoever wishes to be a friend of the world makes himself an enemy of God. Or do you suppose it is to no purpose that the Scripture says, "He yearns jealously over the spirit that he has made to dwell in us? (James 4:1-4)"

What is our enemy trying to control? (You'll find the clue in the first two verses of each passage.)

_____

What are some of the results of the enemy commandeering this aspect of our heart?

_____

What is the enemy's definition of victory? _____

Whatever we ultimately trust for our protection, promotion, and provision, *that* is our god! God's enemy is bitterly jealous of Him. He's also delusional and pathologically ambitious. He wants our worship, but he'll settle for us worshiping anything in the place of worshiping God. Therefore, he works very hard to keep the perception alive that anything other than the One True God is truly trustworthy and will keep us safe. Remember, our brain is DNA programmed to *stay safe*.

Knowing this:

What is the healthiest way to keep our brain safe? _____

Do we want to live guided by a loving brain or the selfish brain? _____

What will be the chemical consequences? _____

Our enemy tries to incite idolatry and selfishness. Most of us would never think of bowing to the devil, but we often find ourselves bowing to our own interests—the "three p's": protection, promotion, and provision. We usually do this through self-protection, self-promotion, self-provision.

Look for four "p" words below and underline them.

> For all that is in the world—the desires of the flesh and the desires of the eyes and pride of life—is not from the Father but is from the world. (1 John 2:16)
>
> I tell you, my friends, do not fear those who kill the body, and after that have nothing more that they can do. But I will warn you whom to fear: fear him who, after he has killed, has authority to cast into hell. Yes, I tell you, fear him! Are not five sparrows sold for two pennies? And not one of them is forgotten before God. Why, even the hairs of your head are all numbered. Fear not; you are of more value than many sparrows. (Luke 12. 4-7)

Ready to get personal? If your luxury car is what brings you the most satisfaction—occupying your thoughts and commanding your resources—it's an idol. If your career is the source of your personal value and validates your existence, it is an idol. If your attractiveness is what you rely on to gain and keep relationships, it's an idol.

An idol is a substitute for God. Seeking an idol for that which only God can righteously provide is idolatry. Pride turns our attention away from our only true source of happiness and health.

What is the enemy's goal for each battle? _____

How does he think he'll win the war? _____

Where is the war fought? _____

In our physical world, wars are between opposing *people*—their will and desire for something, control of resources, ethnic superiority—on material territory. They're fought on the ground, on the water, in the air, and now in cyberspace. Even currency and technology wars are tied to a fight over control of a resource and its superiority.

As we've read from the Bible, the war we're in is for our hearts and minds—our thoughts, wills, and emotions. Our enemy is "not flesh and blood" but rather "rulers", "powers", and "cosmic authorities"—all spiritual beings without human bodies—led by a chief enemy who, although he is also only in spirit form, actively pursues us like a lion seeking a prey.

If the resources to control, and the ideological superiority to gain, are intellectual, volitional, and emotional, the battles will be for our beliefs, for our *will*, and for our *joy*. We may have to fight to do what's right instead of what's expedient. We may have to battle to find joy in what's truly satisfying instead of accepting what passes as pleasure on this earth.

We must also realize that the war for our mind is unrelenting and never-ending. And, if we're not careful, our very health can become a casualty. This realization will help us focus on upshifting our brains to communicate with the One who can create in us a new mind.

WRAPPING IT UP

This may be the first time you've ever read anything about a "spiritual war." It may sound silly, superstitious or unscientific. The gravity of the war and stakes in each battle can create anxiety and fear and activate chemicals, which can destroy us from the inside out.

Remember we're truly living in the mind. Most of our experiences in the real world aren't material; they're in our minds. That's why two people can see the same thing or experience the same thing and be affected very differently, same physical reality, different mental response. We can also influence the physical and material world with our mind. We can stress and elevate our heart rate, blood pressure, and mental acuity. We can choose to be selfish and argue to get an advantage over another person to the point where a physical fight will erupt. Yes, it's in our mind where we live. It's the realm of the intellect, volition, and emotion. It's easy to see how the battle for control is a spiritual battle. Do you understand how important the brain is for health and how are physical choices effect the brain and vice versa?

Ask God to confirm for you whether this is true. Re-read the passages we covered in today's study.

LIVING IN COMMUNITY

Two things bring people together in the most profound ways: love and war. In *Biblical Prescriptions for Life*, we turn to love. Today, you can love your study buddies and fellow students by encouraging them as they move toward healing and wellness on this journey.

You can lock arms with them as you fight together for truth and to stand against the lies that surround us all. Strengthen one another. Help one another identify the strategies and tactics of our enemy. His goal is our destruction.

And keep in mind that, even as you live with your friends and family, there will be inevitable interpersonal conflict. There may be harsh words and tears. But those precious people are NOT your enemy. They are victims, too. The war is *for your mind*.

BECOMING MISSIONAL

This week of study usually brings challenges into life. Why? Because distractions and difficulties can take focus off the real goal. God is changing our beliefs. God is working in your life! If the enemy can discourage you with a sick child, a broken water heater, or a stranded car and get you to give up at this very critical point in your journey, he'll be gaining a foothold.

So, keep your eyes open. Tend to the sick child, fix the water heater, and call a tow truck. But, whatever you do, don't over-spiritualize every circumstance and relationship this week. And while you face the battles we all face, don't disregard the reality of the spiritual war that's taking place for control of your mind. Being missional today means realizing you're in a war.

COMMITMENT

Wars are fought in battles. Some seem insignificant at the time but later are recognized as turning points. Today is a great day to work on your list of *Biblical Prescriptions for Life* action items. And it will be especially beneficial to journal your thoughts as you process the truths we've studied.

Commit yourself to a walk outside with your friends. Drink a bottle of water before you leave. Enjoy a big salad, share some things for which you're thankful, and gift yourself (and others) with a big belly laugh.

Think for a moment, is your understanding of what it takes to be healthy changing? Is this study making sense to you? Is God speaking to your heart?

As your physical self is improving can you hear God better?

DAY 4

The Hopefully Not-So-Secret Weapon

Are you ready for the biggest headline in the cosmos?

"God has Already Won the War for Us; Healing Guaranteed."

In today's lesson, the take home should gladden the heart of every student: The war has been won!

That's right. When God sent His son Jesus to fulfill His perfect plan on our behalf and reconciled us to the Father—this enabled each one of us to have a healthy and growing relationship with the Creator of the Universe. Within this relationship lies the profound realization that the war has already been won!

That brings me to the secret weapon of warfare that the Father has given to each one of us. We, His children, have the *power of choice*. We can *choose* to have Him create in us, a new mind.

Yesterday, we learned that the battle is fought for our mind—our thoughts + will + emotions. A mind tuned to God creates physiological health and spiritual wholeness. The way we use and train our brain is a Biblical Prescription for Life, allowing us to choose to have God create in us a new heart. As I demonstrated in the video session, upshifitng our brains will actually change our brain's chemistry and retrain our neural pathways toward healing.

Science and medicine now has the ability to observe and describe the changes that God told us about in His Word nearly 2,000 years ago. At long last, we have *evidence-based studies and technology* to prove the Word of God.

Read the following passages and mark:

- "Life" and "Spirit of Life" with a simple green leaf

- "Peace", "obedience" and "righteousness" and their synonyms with a green smiley face

- "Desire" and its synonyms with a red heart

- "Flesh" with a black rectangle

- "Death", "lawlessness", "sin" and "condemnation" with a black X

What then? Are we to sin because we are not under law but under grace? By no means! Do you not know that if you present yourselves to anyone as obedient slaves, you are slaves of the one whom you obey, either of sin, which leads to death, or of obedience, which leads to righteousness? But thanks be to God, that you who were once slaves of sin have become obedient from the heart to the standard of teaching to which you were committed, and, having been set free from sin, have become slaves of righteousness. I am speaking in human terms, because of your natural limitations. For just as you once presented your members as slaves to impurity and to lawlessness leading to more lawlessness, so now present your members as slaves to righteousness leading to sanctification. (Romans 6: 15-19)

There is therefore now no condemnation for those who are in Christ Jesus. For the law of the Spirit of life has set you free in Christ Jesus from the law of sin and death. For God has done what the law, weakened by the flesh, could not do. By sending his own Son in the likeness of sinful flesh and for sin, he condemned sin in the flesh, in order that the righteous requirement of the law might be fulfilled in us, who walk not according to the flesh but according to the Spirit. For those who live according to the flesh set their minds on the things of the flesh, but those who live according to the Spirit set their minds on the things of the Spirit. For to set the mind on the flesh is death, but to set the mind on the Spirit is life and peace. For the mind that is set on the flesh is hostile to God, for it does not submit to God's law; indeed, it cannot. Those who are in the flesh cannot please God. (Romans 8:1-8)

Now, make a list of the contrasts we see between the two ways for a child of God to live:

Life in the Spirit   **Life in the Flesh**

_____   _____

_____   _____

_____   _____

_____   _____

_____   _____

_____   _____

_____   _____

How do these two contrasting ways to live affect the physiology of the brain? _____

Read this promise out loud.

> No temptation has overtaken you that is not common to man. God is faithful, and he will not let you be tempted beyond your ability, but with the temptation he will also provide the way of escape, that you may be able to endure it. (1 Corinthians 10:13)

How does this make you feel? _____

In the following passages:

- Mark a green line to underline everything God tells us to do in the war.

- Draw a green rectangle around every promise that relates to our faith-filled obedience.

> For the weapons of our warfare are not of the flesh but have divine power to destroy strongholds. We destroy arguments and every lofty opinion raised against the knowledge of God, and take every thought captive to obey Christ. (2 Corinthians 10:4, 5)

> I appeal to you therefore, brothers, by the mercies of God, to present your bodies as a living sacrifice, holy and acceptable to God, which is your spiritual worship. Do not be conformed to this world, but be transformed by the renewal of your mind, that by testing you may discern what is the will of God, what is good and acceptable and perfect. (Romans 12:1, 2)

> But he gives more grace. Therefore it says, "God opposes the proud, but gives grace to the humble." Submit yourselves therefore to God. Resist the devil, and he will flee from you. Draw near to God, and he will draw near to you. Cleanse your hands, you sinners, and purify your hearts, you double-minded. Be wretched and mourn and weep. Let your laughter be turned to mourning and your joy to gloom. Humble yourselves before the Lord, and he will exalt you. (James 4:6-10)

WRAPPING IT UP

- Is there a real spiritual war?

- Are you and I involved in it?

- On Whose side are we?

- Who has guaranteed our victory?

LIVING IN COMMUNITY

God has given you unfathomable power—*His* power! And He has made you victorious in the battle for your mind. This spiritual power helps every cell in our body.

Making small steps will re-train our neural pathways, one step at a time. This has been our goal with these studies. Now, we can be very helpful to others in the war. You now understand the spiritual realities. You have the skills to strengthen and encourage others as they fight their personal battles in the war.

Be ready—someone may need you very soon.

BEING MISSIONAL

In God's economy, you can do the wrong thing (break your brother's computer) with the right motives (while trying to repair it). God is pleased by your attempt to be loving and helpful. You can also do the right thing (volunteer at the homeless shelter) with the wrong motives (so that others will think better of you) and God will see that as a selfish and unloving act. That said, when people do the right thing for the wrong reasons, that "thing" may still accomplish good in the real world (the homeless are served) and God's love is able to touch their lives. But, for the person who did it with the wrong motives, the benefits are all external—and temporary. While they were a tool that God could use to spread His grace and mercy, they themselves received little to no joy in the presence of the Father.

This week, ask God to help you identify people who need His help. After six weeks of *Biblical Prescriptions for Life*, you have multiple ways to share God's love, health, relationships, and truth. As you serve others, you'll be in a place of worship. Be humble. Be loving. Be a servant. One of the most powerful examples of God's love is the change He's accomplishing in you!

COMMITMENT

Commit yourself to sharing with someone who needs encouragement. Tell him or her what you've learned today. The battle for the mind has been won! We can be anxious about nothing. How are you doing with your nutrition? Remember take it slowly. The brain is involved as well. If you are not happy and your eating stresses you, reassess the situation. The stress caused by your food choices might be doing more harm than good. Look at the big picture! You might need to move slower.

DAY 5

Let's Upshift

God has given us very powerful ways of understanding the spiritual war that's going on all around us. There's a battle for our minds and this affects our health. Our spiritual life and physical well-being are extremely interconnected. This week we've spent time learning some basics about how our brain works. Today we're going to review what we have learned. This will strengthen positive neuropathways.

No one really *wants* to experience illness. Most want to have *healing* in their lives. God will heal everyone who seeks Him. Some He heals dramatically in an instant; others He heals over the long haul through steady change, one step at a time; and everyone He will heal in heaven when there'll be no more sickness or tears. It's not up to any of us in the healing arts to decide which outcome God has for you in this life. But know this—God *will* heal you!

Whatever extent of healing He brings to you, we each have the gift of choice to start the process. I want to return to a key concept I taught in the video session—downshifting and upshifting in the brain.

We learned that the brain could be described in relation to three functional layers with characteristic functions:

1. **Lower brain** (reptilian) . . . . Fight or flight response, survival, core vitals

2. **Mid brain** (mammalian). . . . . . . Memories, emotions, immune system,

3. **Higher brain** (human) . . . . Creativity, relationships, abstract thinking

You can think about *downshift* and *upshift* as both adjectives and verbs.

Downshifted (adjective)	**Upshifted (adjective)**
Alarm reaction mode	Relational, creative, planning mode
Survival mode	Altruistic, loving mode
Downshift/ing (verb)	**Upshift/ing (verb)**
Focusing on selfishness, emotions	Focusing on cognition, the future, relationships
Live in the here and now	Planning and Organizing; delaying gratification
Downshifted Symptoms	**Upshifted Symptoms**
Increase in stress hormones, anxious	Mitigation of stress hormones
Shallow breathing, elevated heart rate	Relaxed, full breathing, lower resting heart rate
Increased blood pressure, inflammation, pain	Rested, clarity, peace
Decreased immune function, decreased cognition	

Unless you're fleeing a burning building or fighting off an attacker, you want to spend your time in the upshifted mode. You want to be a thinker, logical, in a relationship with God. When you find yourself downshifting or in a downshifted mode, recognizing it quickly and taking a few simple actions will help you upshift and return to the upshifted mode.

Let's review how to begin to physiologically upshift:

1. Call it what it is—let yourself recognize you're downshifting or in downshift mode. Understand the physical implications.

2. **Pray** for help from the Ultimate Physician.

3. **Worship.** Next week we will study the importance of worship in upshifitng the brain.

4. **Remember** how God has cared for you in the past.

5. Take **deep breaths.** Release each one fully, from deep in your diaphragm.

6. Remind yourself of five (3) things for which you can be **thankful.**

7. Find something good to **laugh** about.

8. Focus on **being healthy**; water, light, movement, good nutrition.

These are treatments you can apply today!

The following Scripture provides the long-term plan to live more of your life upshifted—in the higher cognition and experiencing life in the Spirit.

The Apostle Paul calls this "putting off" and "putting on" and the word choice is extremely beneficial. That's because God has given us the power to choose where our minds focus. He wants us to choose to stop doing harmful things and start doing healing things!

Mark the following passages this way:

- Every thought, belief and practice that we are told to **put off** with a red rectangle

- Every thought, belief and practice that we are to **put on** with a green rectangle

If then you have been raised with Christ, seek the things that are above, where Christ is, seated at the right hand of God. Set your minds on things that are above, not on things that are on earth. For you have died, and your life is hidden with Christ in God. When Christ who is your life appears, then you also will appear with him in glory.

Put to death therefore what is earthly in you: sexual immorality, impurity, passion, evil desire, and covetousness, which is idolatry. On account of these the wrath of God is coming. In these you too once walked, when you were living in them. But now you must put them all away: anger, wrath, malice, slander, and obscene talk from your mouth. Do not lie to one another, seeing that you have put off the old self with its practices and have put on the new self, which is being renewed in knowledge after the image of its creator.

Put on then, as God's chosen ones, holy and beloved, compassionate hearts, kindness, humility, meekness, and patience, bearing with one another and, if one has a complaint against another, forgiving each other; as the Lord has forgiven you, so you also must forgive.

And above all these put on love, which binds everything together in perfect harmony. And let the peace of Christ rule in your hearts, to which indeed you were called in one body. And be thankful. Let the word of Christ dwell in you richly, teaching and admonishing one another in all wisdom, singing psalms and hymns and spiritual songs, with thankfulness in your hearts to God. And whatever you do, in word or deed, do everything in the name of the Lord Jesus, giving thanks to God the Father through him. (Colossians 3:1-17)

Rejoice in the Lord always; again I will say, rejoice. Let your reasonableness be known to everyone. The Lord is at hand; do not be anxious about anything, but in everything by prayer and supplication with thanksgiving let your requests be made known to God. And the peace of God, which surpasses all understanding, will guard your hearts and your minds in Christ Jesus.

Finally, brothers, whatever is true, whatever is honorable, whatever is just, whatever is pure, whatever is lovely, whatever is commendable, if there is any excellence, if there is anything worthy of praise, think about these things. What you have learned and received and heard and seen in me—practice these things, and the God of peace will be with you. (Philippians 4:4-9)

Now this I say and testify in the Lord, that you must no longer walk as the Gentiles do, in the futility of their minds. They are darkened in their understanding, alienated from the life of God because of the ignorance that is in them, due to their hardness of heart. They have become callous and have given themselves up to sensuality, greedy to practice every kind of impurity. But that is not the way you learned Christ!—assuming that you have heard about him and were taught in him, as the truth is in Jesus, to put off your old self, which belongs to your former manner of life and is corrupt through deceitful desires, and to be renewed in the spirit of your minds, and to put on the new self, created after the likeness of God in true righteousness and holiness.

Therefore, having put away falsehood let each one of you speak the truth with his neighbor, for we are members one of another. Be angry and do not sin; do not let the sun go down on your anger, and give no opportunity to the devil. Let the thief no longer steal, but rather let him labor, doing honest work with his own hands, so that he may have something to share with anyone in need. Let no corrupting talk come out of your mouths, but only such as is good for building up, as fits the occasion, that it may give grace to those who hear. And do not grieve the Holy Spirit of God, by whom you were sealed for the day of redemption. Let all bitterness and wrath and anger and clamor and slander be put away from you, along with all malice. Be kind to one another, tenderhearted, forgiving one another, as God in Christ forgave you. (Ephesians 4:17-32)

Did you know that God had given us clear instructions? I'm so very thankful that I had a teacher who brought me to these passages in the Bible so I could see for myself the things my loving, perfect, heavenly Father wants me to pursue so that I can experience the abundant life He desires for me.

I encourage you to take a moment before we conclude today to record a few key things that God has impressed on you to "put off"—to stop doing; to avoid:

_____

_____

_____

_____

...and to "put on"—to pursue and start doing:

_____

_____

_____

_____

WRAPPING IT UP

God loves you. Like a parent who wants his or her child to be safe, healthy, and to feel loved, our Father wants His best for us.

Take a moment here to thank God in prayer for His perfect, loving plan and His clear instructions. He is so good!

LIVING IN COMMUNITY

In order to be an agent of love and healing in our community—at work, at home, at school, at church, anywhere—we need to follow God's perfect design for life. No, we won't follow it perfectly. We're sinful human beings! So, don't judge yourself or others for failures and setbacks. And don't stop moving forward! When you fail, talk to God about it. Ask for forgiveness. Ask for power to start again. And then trust Him with the next step of love you take.

When someone fails you, extend them the same grace. Living in a community of people following Jesus moves us all in the same direction toward healing and whole-life, life-long wellness. It is about direction, not perfection. Christ has extended grace to make up for our shortcomings. It begins in our mind and flows out through our choices. It's a Biblical Prescription for Life.

BEING MISSIONAL

One way we move forward on mission is by protecting the vulnerable from the harm of sin. If you know someone who is hurting others by their choices, you may need to wisely and gently intervene—first through private prayer, then with the appropriate partners (people who love them and want the best for them while desiring to protect the vulnerable from harm). Don't go at it alone.

COMMITMENT

What have you learned about your inner life—the life of your mind—this week through your journaling? As we said, you are the person you listen to most. That's one more reason why healthy, healing, Godward thoughts are a Biblical Prescription for Life.

Take some time to breathe deeply. Take a slow, deep breathe, hold for three seconds, and exhale ever so slowly and repeat this ten times. Some may want to breathe this way for up to ten minutes. Deep breathing is a relaxing response and turns down the sympathetic nervous system, which generates the stress response and turns up the parasympathetic nervous system that counteracts the stress chemistry. When we are stressed we become shallow breathers. Breathing deeply also helps the brain chemistry upshift, not only by turning down stress chemistry, but by improving oxygen, relaxing muscles, and focusing thoughts. Try this activity now and incorporate this relaxation response when you feel you are downshifting.

—— DAY 6 ——————————————

Brain Toxin

As we've been learning this week, we must strive to optimize the function of our pre-frontal cortex. Upshifting the brain is very important, but there are toxins in our world, which damage the brain and make upshifting difficult or even impossible. Alcohol and drugs like cocaine, heroin, and methamphetamines cause the brain to function sub-optimally. Prescription medication can also change the brain's functioning.

Of course, there are physical factors like not getting enough rest, lack of oxygen, dehydration and a lack of nutrients. I want to focus today's lesson on the less obvious toxins. Remember, all inputs are processed in the brain. Those inputs will either be harmful or beneficial. They will either cause stress leading to downshifting or help the brain upshift. This is important because our communication with God occurs in the neocortex, the new brain. A damaged brain will have more stress and will downshift as it tries to keep itself "safe," thus making it more difficult to communicate with God.

Since Edison came along and invented the light bulb, our brains have been working more after dark. Before the light bulb we use to go to bed at night. Now we are in a 24/7 never ending cycle. Our natural rhythms—our circadian rhythms—have been disrupted causing stress. So not only do we have toxic inputs flooding in, we now can have them flooding in longer and longer each day. That's not a good thing!

I want to focus for a moment on all the inputs that arrive in our brain from a very popular source: the media.

Does exposure to media stress the brain? A Ball State University study released in 2006 pointed out that the average adult spends 9 hours a day with various forms of media. This would include watching television (6 hours) or using a computer, (2 hours). But that was just the beginning. In 2008, just two years later, it's been estimated that the total time spent each day on media was 635 minutes. That's over 10 hours! In 2009 that number eased up to 650 minutes/day and in 2010 660 minutes/day were spent per person. Notice the trend. Every year, more and more brain input was coming from the media, and, while the majority of this time was spent with television and Internet, mobile devices were trending upward at a rapid pace.

Let's follow that journey:

2010

- 4 hours and 20 minutes a day on TV and video

- 2 hours and 35 minutes online

- 50 minutes a day on other devices

2012

- 4 hours and 15 minutes with television

- 4.58 hours online

- 2.88 hours on mobile devices

Notice the increase of time spent on mobile devices. More time is still spent on television than any other form of media, but the uses of newer media devices (mobile phones, tablets, computers, etc.) are increasing while older media like television, newspapers, magazines and radio are decreasing. The bottom line is: we spend much of our lives receiving inputs from the media. So, how are these constant inputs changing our brains?

When we see violence, bad news, clinically disturbing rhetoric, or anything that induces a stress response, our brain must handle that input. It also must *balance* the input.

The right brain is the divergent thinking section. It's more imaginative, intuitive and abstract. It tends to work holistically, integrating pieces of information into a whole.

The left-brain is for convergent thinking and processes information logically and analytically but lacks the "big picture" ability. The left-brain works out the details of life. The right brain helps us understand the reason why.

The right hemisphere also integrates our belief systems and appreciates music and art. If we see a ball at a baseball game, the left-brain tells us, "Hey, that's a ball." The right brain tells us, "Hey, that ball is used to play the game and here's how."

Balance between the left and right hemispheres is critical. When it's disrupted, stress ensues. And here's the bad news. The media disrupts this balance because the left-brain is stimulated much more than the right.

Seven studies have now confirmed that babies who watch television have delayed language development. The average American 18-year-old has witnessed 200,000 acts of violence, 15,000 sexual acts, and 2,000 beer and wine commercials in their lifetime. Needless to say, this is stressing the brain on many levels. In 2007, Frederick Zimmerman, writing in the Journal Pediatrics (November 2007, 120 5 986-992), reported that violent or nonviolent programming caused attention problems while purely educational programs did not.

Here is another interesting set of data. The murder rate in South Africa from 1945-1974 declined 17%. During those very same years, the murder rate in the US and UK increased by 93% and 92% respectively. Those were years when the US saw television take-off. When television was introduced to South Africa in 1974, murder rates rose 30% higher from 1974-1987. Coincidence? I don't think so.

The preceding evidence suggests that the media, as a whole, is damaging brains and diminishing our world's ability to communicate with our Creator. I consider the media as a whole to be a brain toxin, perhaps the most damaging element ever to our brain. It's a subtle but effective downshifter. Remember stress causes physical changes, which, in time, cause symptoms and altered physiology. Brain inputs to the health are just as important, if not more, than the stress that comes from not moving or eating the wrong foods. Technology still has not explained the complexities of the brain and the physiologic effects. However, we know rates of anxiety are rising. Many have mental health problems. The rates are rising. There has to be a cause. God admonishes to be anxious about nothing and wants us not to fear. God knew that brain inputs would be a problem for His children. However, there is encouraging news.

There's much we can do—one step at a time—to improve brain function. How can we begin making progress? Knowing that the brain works best with positives is a good start. This is very important. One positive is to strive to spend less time with media. Also, we can all honestly evaluate whether the media we're ingesting is toxic to our brain.

Learn and find ways to improve

The practice of keeping a journal is very helpful. As you track how you spend time, you begin to discover recurring themes that reveal deeply travelled neural pathways—some healthful, some harmful.

The key is journal honestly. Your journal is just for you and God. Don't hide anything. Don't stop when you get bored or start to lose resolve. In fact, in those days, you may find some great illumination! Sometimes, we know we're headed for an old habit and we stop journaling so that we can hide that fact a little easier. We stop so we don't have to confront the harmful beliefs with which we've become comfortable.

Remember where we started with *Biblical Prescriptions for Life*? We committed to be honest and address the hard topics even if they made us uncomfortable. Remember Jesus' question to the paralyzed man at the Pool of Bethsaida—"Do you want to be made well?" I hope you do. I *know* I do. If you've let it slide, why not dust yourself off and start journaling with raw honesty.

Did you discover that you're holding onto brain inputs that are harmful? If you did, then journaling is doing its job!

The key is to ask your study buddy or small group to help you find promises straight from God's word that address those harmful inputs that will eventually have an impact on your brain. Call them in your moment of weakness. We heal best in community.

Return to Walking in the Light

If you find yourself out of sync with health, it's important to understand where and why you left the path of healing. Then call it out for what it was. That act is what we called confession or "agreeing with God" in the lesson on light. If it was doubt, confess your doubt to God and ask Him for faith to trust Him and gain the power to overcome. If you gave in to the temptation for a momentary pleasure, confess it. "I overate," or "I was angry at my sister." God forgives and throws our shortcomings into the sea. We need to do the same. Do not replay shortcomings. Do not relive yesterday. Live today with God the best you can. Doing this will help you realize that you don't have to provide for, promote, or protect yourself.

This is a great time to revisit God's way back to the light, found in 1 John.

> If we confess our sins, He is faithful and just to forgive us our sins and to cleanse us from all unrighteousness. (1 John 1:9)

What a promise to us who confess and repent! Thank God for His mercy and grace!

Put off and Put on

In week two of *Biblical Prescriptions for Life*, we kept track of our drink choices. This week we listed our media choices. I was shocked at the time I was spending on the media. I can do better. I didn't realize my problem until I asked God to help me. As I've learned the critical importance of the brain and my thoughts, I want God to help create in me a new brain to have a better relationship with Him. This includes evaluating media choices. In some instances I didn't realize I was working against myself and arming the enemy as he tried to take control of my mind.

If you find yourself stuck, I encourage you to journal your media consumption. Use this chart for a week and pray about what you learn. Be honest. And then take action..

Media & minutes consumed	The specific message	The result—upshift or downshift?

Don't judge yourself. Do judge the media's messages.

Hold your brain accountable

Biblical Prescriptions for Life exposes us to new truths in ways we may have not experienced before. Examining the spiritual content of media inputs opens awareness to the life of our mind that we may have previously overlooked or minimized.

Try to focus on positives while moving forward. However, it can be very helpful when we find ourselves stuck to look more closely at our behavior—situation, motivation, and results—so that we can face them in the light of honest truth. Harmful habits survive because of harmful underlying beliefs. Let's pull those out into the light where we can deal with them. This worksheet may be helpful for us.

What I did: _____

Who was I focused on? _____

What was I focused on before I did it? _____

Where was I when I decided to act? _____

When did I act—what time of day? Was I tired? Was I alone? Was I bored? Was I angry?

_____

Why did I choose to act? What benefit did I think I'd get from my action this time? And why did I think it would be helpful and healing to act this way on this occasion as opposed to earlier times?

_____

_____

What will give/restore peace and pleasure? _____

Will it be enduring, good pleasure for which I give thanks to God, or will it be a short term fix that will leave me ashamed, in a deeper hold, filled with regrets, stress and relational damage?

_____

Looking back, can I spot when I made the downshift? Fear, shame, and thoughtless desire usually put me in the mode where I focus on becoming my own protector, promoter, and provider. I become selfish, not selfless.

_____

Who can help me get unstuck? Put a person's name here that you will share this struggle with and ask for help.

_____

Stay Holistic

God created us with beautiful, complex, integrated bodies. Yes, we can talk in terms of systems—cardiovascular, pulmonary, central nervous, gastrointestinal, etc.—but scientists are now learning and starting to acknowledge the truths that God revealed at the beginning. We're an integrated mind, body and spirit.

Let's run through the basics from Lessons 1-5:

1. Are you drinking water?

2. Are you breathing deeply?

3. Are you getting out into the sunlight?

4. Are you moving—walking, exercising?

5. Are you converting more of your diet to a plant-based, whole food diet?

6. And from this week's lesson: Are you maximizing brain function? Do you have an upshifting strategy?

WRAPPING IT UP

We've learned that in God's power and with our hopeful choices, we have the power to transform our lives. I can't say enough about what the God of the universe can do to bring healing into our lives. Brain inputs just like food inputs have physiological consequences. The media is now a major source of input. Is the media stressing your brain causing a subtle downshifting of function?

LIVING IN COMMUNITY

Sometimes we need someone to ask us, "How are you doing?" and then lovingly wait for the _true_ answer.

You've been in meaningful community with your study buddy and small group for nearly six full weeks now. If you've followed Biblical Prescriptions for Life, you might be experiencing some of the deepest relationships you've enjoyed in years. It may be time to take it to the next level. If you sense someone in your group is stuck, offer to be used by God as a lifeline to help them get unstuck.

BECOMING MISSIONAL

Your small group is a valid place to be missional. Your family is a great place to be missional. Any place where you can have a meaningful conversation is a great place to reach out with God's love, hope, and healing.

Jesus used health as one of His primary means to reach the hurting and spiritually seeking. You'll find people will open up about their health with very little effort. Sharing the transformation God is accomplishing in your life is an authentic way to open a communication channel about the Great Physician. But, don't rush it. Don't try to cover all the ground in one conversation. Also, never shy away when God gives you the green light to say something in love. He'll provide the words to say.

COMMITMENT

Charge that battery 1. For yourself, 2. For your study buddy, 3. And for the person with whom God leads you to share in the near future.

Take the time to again evaluate how the media is changing your brain.

Commit to steps to improve and limit, if necessary, these inputs. Just like the other changes we have made, move one step at a time with the Ultimate Physician holding your hand along the journey.

DAY 7

Worship Our Victorious King

As you enter your day of rest this week—a very important Biblical Prescription for Life—here are a few prompts that will hopefully tune your heart and mind to faith, gladness, and thankfulness. These are powerful expressions of authentic worship.

- The Kingdom of Light is God's Kingdom. He owns it. He rules it in complete love. He rules it with the power of His word. He cannot be defeated, challenged or fatigued.

- We are citizens of His Kingdom by His invitation. He sustains us by His favor. His gives us victory over any vestiges of darkness in our old beliefs and habits by His power. No one can take us from His Kingdom. We are safe.

- He will complete the good work He has begun in us, turning us from darkness to light. Saving us from the curse of selfish rebellion to the covenant of love. Healing us. Satisfying us.

- The war is real. But God is more than strong enough to fight it for us

This is the historical account of one of the times the Israelites were under siege by the Syrians.

> Once when the king of Syria was warring against Israel, he took counsel with his servants, saying, "At such and such a place shall be my camp." But the man of God sent word to the king of Israel, "Beware that you do not pass this place, for the Syrians are going down there." And the king of Israel sent to the place about which the man of God told him. Thus he used to warn him, so that he saved himself there more than once or twice.
>
> And the mind of the king of Syria was greatly troubled because of this thing, and he called his servants and said to them, "Will you not show me who of us is for the king of Israel?" And one of his servants said, "None, my lord, O king; but Elisha, the prophet who is in Israel, tells the king of Israel the words that you speak in your bedroom." And he said, "Go and see where he is, that I may send and seize him." It was told him, "Behold, he is in Dothan." So he sent there horses and chariots and a great army, and they came by night and surrounded the city.
>
> When the servant of the man of God rose early in the morning and went out, behold, an army with horses and chariots was all around the city. And the servant said, "Alas, my master! What shall we do?" He said, "Do not be afraid, for those who are with us are more than those who are with them." Then Elisha prayed and said, "O Lord, please open his eyes that he may see." So the Lord opened the eyes of the young man, and he saw, and behold, the mountain was full of horses and chariots of fire all around Elisha. (2 Kings 6:8-17)

The war was real. The soldiers were real. The danger was real and imminent. In God's kindness to Elisha's servant, He showed him a glimpse into the spiritual reality to give him peace in the presence of Israel's enemy.

May God give us peace. He has guaranteed the victory. We will be made well! Trust God for healing.

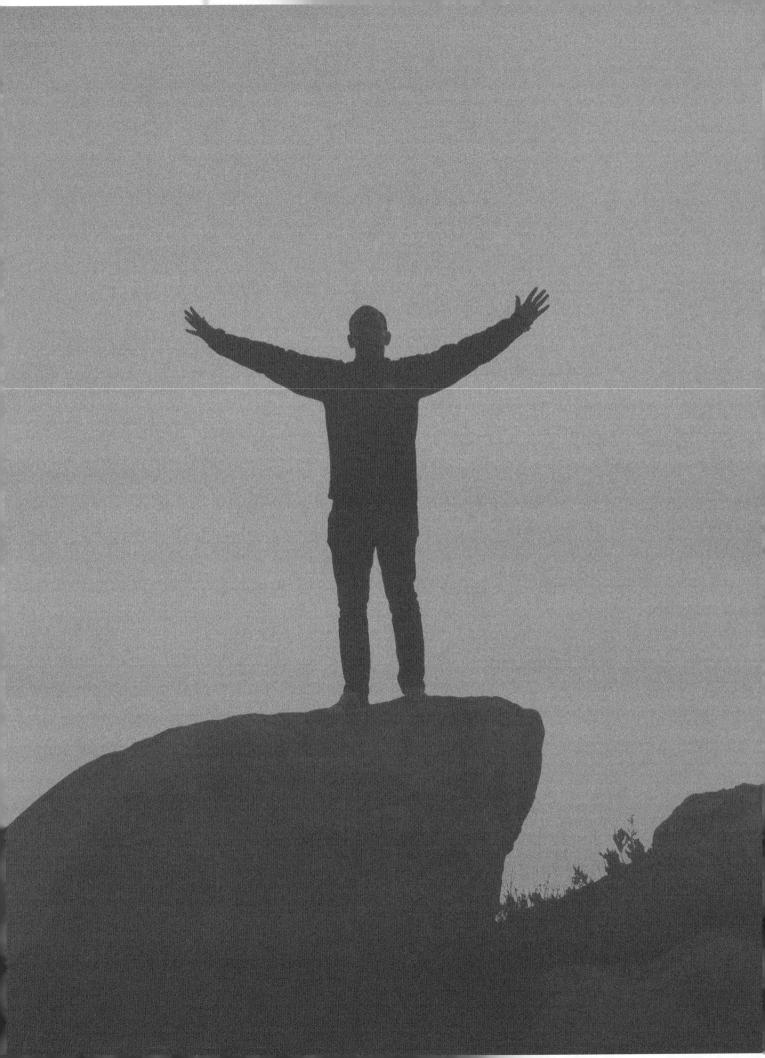

WEEK 7

Biblical Prescription for Life 6—Worship

Tom was a successful businessman, father, and husband. One day while at work, he suddenly felt as if an elephant had sat down on his chest. He'd never experienced this sensation before.

Understandably, Tom was scared and immediately sought help. He dialed 911 and soon found himself being ushered into the emergency room of a nearby hospital. It didn't take doctors long to diagnose that he'd suffered a myocardial infarction (blood flow stopped to part of the heart) and Tom quickly received a stent to re-open his right coronary artery. Fortunately, his care had come quickly enough to escape permanent heart damage. This was modern medicine at its best!

That event, striking him in his mid-thirties, left him petrified. From that point on, any time he felt "off" in his chest, he panicked. He regularly visited doctors, hurried to emergency rooms and endured extensive testing on his heart. He saw doctor after doctor, trying to find a reason for his very real symptoms. Tom needed help!

His cardiologists examined the repeated tests and offered reassurance that all was well, but it wasn't. His psychologist did everything he could in the cognitive therapy world and determined that all was well there too, but it wasn't. Tom ate healthy, exercised, took time off from work, but nothing seemed to help.

At long last, Tom did find healing, but it wasn't at the hospital, on the psychologist's couch, at the dinner table, or on the jogging course. You may find this hard to believe, but Tom healed his ongoing pain through worship.

We've discussed brain function and alluded to worship as a healing modality. This week we'll review the science of worship and discover evidence that it actually changes the body dramatically. Worship, it seems, is a treatment. It's a gift that's different for each individual but the results are the same. Worship heals.

I spent time teaching Tom about the anterior cingulate cortex and the steps to take when symptoms occurred. He learned the difference between acute stress and chronic stress. But as Tom learned about worship, his chest pains finally began to improve. When we added worship to his treatment regimen, his life changed.

This week we'll study worship in a manner that may be new to you. We'll discover that it's a way to fight aging and treat every chronic disease condition known to us.

You may not realize it, but we've already begun the healing journey that worship offers. We've been worshiping every day of this series and have been enjoying the health benefits. Now, in our final week, we'll tie the lessons together and build a sustainable framework for the future.

Understanding water, light, movement, nutrition, the brain and ways to combat stress are all necessary ingredients to help us maximize our worship. Continuing along those lines, I want to emphasize the different ways that worship is a valuable treatment. Restful worship provides balance and helps us deal with the stress chemistry of life. You'll see what I mean when we examine the evidence.

Tom never dreamed that worship would be the key treatment for his symptoms. Modern medicine served an important role when he was having a heart attack, but was not able to quantify or label the current problem. But, as we're discovering, when we delve into God's complex creation and return to His original plan for us, the health benefits are inevitable. Worship was and is part of that plan.

In worship, God reveals Himself to us. Why? Without God in our lives, we experience the stress of uncertainty and a dangerous loss of hope. We were made to be with God. We were made to worship God. When we worship our Creator, there are changes in physiology. Stress chemistry is reduced. Science is just beginning to understand the process.

Let me ask a question: are you resting enough?

"Resting?" I hear you say. "Are you kidding me? Who has time? I'm going 24/7! I have to stay up late just to get everything done and then I have to hit the road early for my job. There are schedules to keep, kids to transport, and preparations to be made for the next busy day. Don't talk to me about resting."

Herein lies the problem. Rest and worship are joined at the hip. You really can't enjoy the full benefits of one without the other.

Let's take a closer look at rest. What is it to you? Is it sleeping at night? Perhaps sitting down in a chair is rest. Well, you're on the right track. Our bodies were designed to rest, to have "down time" on a regular basis. Why is this important? Because every part of us needs rest. It's an absolute requirement. There is more than the physical rest. We need mental rest as well as spiritual rest.

If you broke your arm throwing fastballs, you wouldn't keep throwing fastballs. If you were sick to the stomach, you wouldn't keep right on eating. If your brain is exhausted, do you go looking for complex math problems to solve? Our designer built us to rest. As a matter of fact, His original plan was for us to work during the day and, when the sun goes down, to rest. We were not designed to rest all the time. There was work to do, but balance was vital.

At night, our chemistry changes. Our circadian rhythms kick in. Our entire physiology slows down. Then, when the sun comes back up again, our body revs up to face another day. Rest time is over. That's how we were designed. But how many of us are actually following that divine plan?

In the 1950s, if someone had a heart attack, bed rest was frequently prescribed and we still prescribe it to this day. If you stop and think about it, this makes sense. We rest our agitated gastrointestinal system by not eating. We rest our overworked cardiovascular system by lessening demands on it. When my son broke a bone in his hand, the doctor forced it to "rest" by immobilizing his hand in a cast.

But, in our modern day world, rest is in short supply. We've got the lights on 24/7. The media is constantly bombarding us with messages that our brains instinctively work to analyze. Our neighbors keep upping the ante with their latest purchase and we've got to work harder just to keep up. Technology requires us to relearn everything every few years. Rest—and its close companion, worship—is daily sacrificed on the altar of need and greed. Without proper rest, stress ensues. Healing on all levels slows.

I hope you're getting the picture. That's why I want to review different types of rest to discover where we may be deficient. There's:

- Physical rest (healing the body)

- Mental rest (healing the mind)

- Spiritual rest (healing our relationship with God)

Now consider this amazing passage from God's Holy Word. Why not commit it to memory right now?

> Come to me, all who labor and are heavy laden, and I will give you rest. (Matthew 11:28).

Do you remember this text from week one? In these words I hear God saying, "Listen all you who are burdened by life. Come to me. Worship me. Be with me. And I will provide what your mind, body, and soul need most: beautiful, rejuvenating, healing *rest*!"

This week we'll learn how worship changes the chemistry and brings rest to the body. We have come full circle in our study: from the cause of disease (stress) to the solution (rest). The preceding weeks have helped us optimize the function of our bodies in order to maximize our worship. Now we can prepare to learn how to better receive that gift. May God be with each one of us as we learn about and better apply the treatment of rest.

VIDEO GUIDE 7

Worship and Rest

Key verses:

- Mathew 11:28
- Daniel 6:10-12, 25-27
- 2 Timothy 1:7
- 1 John 4:18
- 1 John 4:8
- Psalm 100

Think about Tom and answer these questions:

1. What do you think he was like before his heart attack? _____

2. How was his life at work? _____

3. How do you think he related to his family? _____

4. What do you think he enjoyed doing in his spare time? _____

Now, answer those same questions to reflect Tom's condition *after* the heart attack but *before* he discovered worship.

1. _____

2. _____

3. _____

4. _____

Can you think of times in your life when your body had problems and the doctor found nothing wrong? Write it down here: _____

What do you think were the main teaching points in the video?

1. _____

2. _____

3. _____

Think back to our previous weeks. Write down at least one main point you remember from each lesson. I'll provide some clues.

1. (Michelle and her stress) _____

2. (H2O) _____

3. (Not inside) _____

4. (Keep moving!) _____

5. (You are what you...) _____

6. (Upshifing) _____

Write down your definition of "rest": _____

Group discussion (20 minutes)

Thinking about worship and rest:

- How can the physical changes you've made during the last few weeks alter the way you worship?_____

- How are your physical health and spirituality connected? _____

- Can you be healthy in one area and not the other? _____

LIVING IN COMMUNITY

Form several groups and each choose one of these texts. Discuss how these texts relate to worship and then share your conclusion with the whole group.

- Acts 6 (The story of Stephen)

- Daniel 6:10-12, 25-27 (Daniel's worship experience)

- Psalm 100 (David and worship)

INDIVIDUAL REFLECTION

Ask yourself: "In my life, is my worship resulting in rest? Do I really understand the types of rest?" Be honest and record your responses here: _____

BEING MISSIONAL

Write down a name for whom to specifically:

- Pray for this week:_____

- Introduce to the power of worship: _____

- Teach about the types of rest: _____

COMMITMENT

Commit these beautiful texts to memory:

- 2 Timothy 1:7

- 1 John 4:18

- 1 John 4:8

Remember, to begin to know God we must worship God and enjoy the gift of His rest.

DAY 1

Physiology of Worship

After his heart attack, Tom continued to have chest pains without knowing the cause. After a thorough evaluation, it was felt that inflammation and an increased load of stress chemicals could be generating his symptoms. As is often the case, once a patient knows what's causing his or her symptoms, they begin to feel better. It was the same with Tom. He thought he was going "crazy." I assured him he wasn't and that the symptoms were originating in his mind as a result of stress.

As you recall from our study of the brain, Tom was definitely *downshifted*. He was over-reacting to his pain and jumping to the conclusion that he was experiencing another heart attack. Although he was right to be concerned, he was making matters worse by allowing his muscles to become tight and inflamed from the stress chemicals. The higher functioning brain would not let him logically sort through whether the symptoms were life threatening or not. His emotional brain insisted they were, and he downshifted.

I directed Tom to Mathew 11:28. He needed to come unto Jesus and he needed to do it right away. I think it's sad that, when we face uncertainty, the last place many of us turn is to the Savior.

I also introduced Tom to the work of Dr. Andrew Newberg. Dr. Newberg has done research on the physiology of worship. Using an amazing device—a PET scanner—he studied the brains of people who take time to commune with their God. Those who worshiped a mere twelve minutes a day were changing the circuitry of the brain in just a few months. Not only were the neurons and connections rearranging themselves, but also stress chemistry was decreasing while chemicals like dopamine and GABA—helpful, healing chemicals—were on the rise! Physical changes in the brain were noted when scans before worship and after worship were compared.

One more noteworthy discovery must be included. Those positive changes occurred in individuals who worshiped what they considered to be a loving, benevolent God.

Dr. Newberg's book, "How God Changes Your Brain," offers much more detail, but the bottom line is abundantly clear: worshiping a loving God for a mere twelve minutes a day for two months changes the brain. Just think what more worship can do. How about a lifetime of worship?

This makes me think of Enoch. Enoch was the father of Methuselah and the Old Testament presents him as a man who "walked with God" (Genesis 5:22). I'd love to sit down and talk with him about his time on Earth—and his "walk." The root word used here is "halak" and can be described as a "movement." This root can also mean movement as in "behavior." So Enoch walked with his mind and behavior in tune with God. He did this for 365 years.

I don't know about you, but in our Matthew text, I hear God saying to me, " Come walk with me, worship me, behave as my spirit moves your mind."

Through Dr. Newberg's work, we're just beginning to comprehend the neuro-physiologic consequences of walking with God. These processes are very complicated, but there's a physical reason why churchgoers enjoy a 30-35% reduced risk of death.

On the flip side, I need to mention what I believe are the consequences to the physiology when we do *not* walk with God.

As I've stated before, we're genetically wired to have a loving relationship with our Creator. When this is not happening, stress is provoked at some level. Dr. Newberg demonstrated how worship increases the development of the higher parts of the brain: the pre-frontal cortex and the anterior cingulate cortex. Knowing what we know, I'd love to study the brains of those who do not worship the true God. The end goal is for us to be like Enoch and walk with God and be close to God through worship.

After I reviewed the evidence-based science with Tom and he read Dr. Newberg's book, he began to worship. He began to spend time with the Creator—to walk with God in a new and dynamic way. That's when his symptoms began to improve. His epinephrine and cytokine levels began to decrease leading to less inflammation, less tightness in his pectoral muscles. I explained that the physiologic benefits of worship on brain physiology is much more complicated. But, getting to know God on a personal level leads to love and a future while non-worship—or worshiping non-benevolent gods—leads to stress and a focus on the present and not on the future. Science is beginning to explain the health benefits of God's words. Many of God's words do not have the scientific studies that explain their benefits—yet. But now that we have brain imaging and can map changes in gene activation, I suspect more and more studies will demonstrate the science of God's words. Even though our current understanding is limited. God's word is true and the laws of the universe are constant. His words support His creation.

Read the following texts and circle the words that you believe would help bring healing to your mind and body through worship:

> God is our refuge and strength, a very present help in trouble. Therefore will not we fear, though the earth be removed, and though the mountains be carried into the midst of the sea. (Psalm 46:1,2)
>
> The Lord is my rock, and my fortress, and my deliverer; my God, my strength, in whom I will trust; my buckler, and the horn of my salvation, and my high tower. (Psalm 18:2)
>
> He gives power to the faint, and to him who has no might he increases strength. (Isaiah 40:29)
>
> Be strong, and let your heart take courage, all you who wait for the Lord! (Psalm 31:24)

Worshiping God is the ultimate upshifting that we can enjoy each and every day. Determine right now that you're going to start making time with God during your busy day. Write down your new "God Time" and don't let anything stand in your way. Complete this sentence:

I promise myself that I will spend _____ minutes each day in worship and communion with God.

I'll do this by: _____

WRAPPING IT UP

Bottom line: We now have scientific evidence that supports the concept of how worshiping changes our physiology and even our DNA. But be warned. Worship has a few side effects to consider. It can lead to a peaceful thought, a hopeful attitude, a forgiving spirit, and most profound of all, a healthier body.

Thinking back on what we've learned, study this list of brain chemicals and write + or – if you think it increases or decreases with prolonged worship.

- ❏   Endorphin (reduces our perception of pain)

- ❏   Cortisol (helps put body in "fight or flight" mode)

- ❏   Inflammatory cytokines (initiate responses against infection)

- ❏   Epinephrine (speeds up the heart and constricts blood vessels, makes muscles tighten)

- ❏   Oxytocin (produces a feeling of love and satisfaction)

- ❏   Dopamine (makes you feel and do happy things)

LIVING IN COMMUNITY

This is the last week together as a group.

- •   Take time to let the group members know how much you appreciate them.

- •   Write a letter to the group and plan on sharing it aloud at the end of the week.

- •   Pray for each other after making a prayer list.

Be honest and open with the other members. Let them know that you'd appreciate their prayers on these two aspects of your life.

1. _____

2. _____

Remember, there's power in prayer!

BEING MISSIONAL

I hope you found today's lesson on the physiology of worship encouraging. Why not find someone in your circle of friends that you can encourage to enjoy the healing benefits of worship? Invite them to participate in some type of worship with you. This isn't about judgment or organized religion. It's about living in line with the Creator's ideal for us all. In whatever way you choose to worship, ask a friend to join you if appropriate.

COMMITMENT

Have you been continuing the changes we've learned about week after week? Are you:

- Walking outside?

- Drinking enough water (half your body weight in ounces)?

- Eating great, health-promoting foods? (That would be plant foods, right?)

- De-stressing your brain with worship?

Never too late to start! Practice makes perfect!

As we move through this week, pray about starting a study with a new group of friends who need this information, who need the relationship with Jesus. This is spreading the Gospel!

—— DAY 2 ——

When Stones Fly

Did you think, as you were doing the last six lessons, that you were changing your physiology while worshipping?

The Biblical Prescriptions of water, light, movement, good nutrition, and a healthy brain alter the physiology of every cell in your body. They've been busy lowering stress levels, allowing you to avoid aging, turning off the expression of damaging genes, and—most importantly—enhancing worship.

Remember how our lessons supported a physical and a spiritual truth? Here's a quick review:

Drinking water is vital to the physiology of our body just as God's "Living Water" brings healing to our souls.

Movement increases muscle tone and circulation while enjoying a "spiritual walk" with God enhances our enjoyment of life itself.

Good nutrition makes present life sustainable just as the "Bread of Life" makes future life possible.

Being outside and receiving **sunlight** delivers a multitude of benefits while the "Light of Truth" generates everlasting joys.

Rest is important to every cell and worship brings about amazing adjustments to our brains.

Today, I want to start with one of the Bible stories that inspires me most. After Christ's ascension, the early Christian church struggled for a foothold in a not-so-welcoming society. This is when we meet someone by the name of Stephen.

> Now Stephen, a man full of God's grace and power, performed great wonders and signs among the people. Opposition arose, however, from members of the Synagogue of the Freedmen (as it was called)—Jews of Cyrene and Alexandria as well as the provinces of Cilicia and Asia—who began to argue with Stephen. But they could not stand up against the wisdom the Spirit gave him as he spoke.
>
> Then they secretly persuaded some men to say, "We have heard Stephen speak blasphemous words against Moses and against God."
>
> So they stirred up the people and the elders and the teachers of the law. They seized Stephen and brought him before the Sanhedrin. They produced false witnesses, who testified, "This fellow never stops speaking against this holy place and against the law. For we have heard him say that this Jesus of Nazareth will destroy this place and change the customs Moses handed down to us."
>
> All who were sitting in the Sanhedrin looked intently at Stephen, and they saw that his face was like the face of an angel. (Acts 6:8-15)

When members of the Sanhedrin asked Stephen if the accusations were true, the man presented them with a history lesson, revealing in vivid details how their ancestors had repeatedly rejected God's leading and message of love. He then looked them right in the eyes and said:

> "You are just like your ancestors: You always resist the Holy Spirit! Was there ever a prophet your ancestors did not persecute? They even killed those who predicted the coming of the Righteous One. And now you have betrayed and murdered him— you who have received the law that was given through angels but have not obeyed it" (verses 51-53).

The reaction of those Stephen was addressing was swift and violent.

> When the members of the Sanhedrin heard this, they were furious and gnashed their teeth at him. But Stephen, full of the Holy Spirit, looked up to heaven and saw the glory of God, and Jesus standing at the right hand of God. "Look," he said, "I see heaven open and the Son of Man standing at the right hand of God."
>
> At this they covered their ears and, yelling at the top of their voices, they all rushed at him, dragged him out of the city and began to stone him. Meanwhile, the witnesses laid their coats at the feet of a young man named Saul.
>
> While they were stoning him, Stephen prayed, "Lord Jesus, receive my spirit." Then he fell on his knees and cried out, "Lord, do not hold this sin against them." When he had said this, he fell asleep (verses 54-60).

Talk about a stressful situation! But, notice how Stephen, throughout the ordeal and even to the painful and violent end, remained in a state of worship. His testimony to the council was clear and concise. Even when facing death, his soul was at rest. I have tears come to my eyes when I wonder how the religious leaders could be so heartless. What were Stephen's friends and family feeling?

Stephen is an example for all ages of what the Holy Spirit can accomplish if we live in an attitude of worship. If I could have measured that man's endorphins and oxytocin levels, I'm sure they would have been off the charts. He loved those who were harming him.

I don't know about you, but I want this type of restful spirit. Stephen didn't overreact or take things personally. He trusted God to take care of him as he witnessed to the world. He had peace in the face of a storm. He allowed God to accomplish His will in his life.

Stephen lived life in an attitude of worship and filled with the Holy Spirit, serving the early church as best he could. And while doing so, he wore "the face of an angel".

In talking with patients, I emphasize rest. In Stephen's case, we saw a soul at rest. He engendered spiritual rest, a peace of mind, allowing a higher power to keep him focused on others, not self. In him, we see a man growing his anterior cingulate cortex and not allowing his amygdyla to control him.

This allowed him (as described in Acts 7:60) to cry out for all to hear: "Lord, do not hold this sin against them." Wow. The Holy Spirit and his worship of the true God had transformed Stephen. Because of this, he carried so much love in his heart. The higher functions of his brain were so strong that the sin-programmed physiology to fight back or run away was completely overpowered. His worship had altered his brain to the point that he could love those who were going to take his life.

Does all this sound familiar to you? Allow me to share a couple verses from a scene from another man's life that was also facing death at the hands of angry liars.

> When they came to the place called the Skull, they crucified him there, along with the criminals—one on his right, the other on his left. Jesus said, "Father, forgive them, for they do not know what they are doing."
>
> It was now about noon, and darkness came over the whole land until three in the afternoon, for the sun stopped shining. And the curtain of the temple was torn in two. Jesus called out with a loud voice, "Father, into your hands I commit my spirit." When he had said this, he breathed his last. (Luke 23:33, 34, 44-46)

Living in an attitude of worship was Christ's most powerful weapon against evil, too.

We've covered the fact that the cells of the body need down time; that those circadian rhythms (the day-night cycle) are there for a reason. But, according to the Bible, there's another cycle of which we need to be aware. It's not daily. It's weekly.

Sabbath rest, as introduced during Creation Week, also plays an important role in our health and well-being. Consider this verse. It's one of the Ten Commandments God offered to the Children of Israel.

Circle the words with red ink that form the requirements for that rest and put a blue square around those whom God wants to benefit from keeping this important and often overlooked commandment.

> Remember the Sabbath day by keeping it holy. Six days you shall labor and do all your work, but the seventh day is the Sabbath to the lord your God. On it you shall not do any work, neither you, nor your son or daughter, nor your manservant or maidservant, not your animals, nor the alien within your gates. For in six days the Lord made the heavens and the earth, the sea, and all that is in them, but he rested on the seventh day. Therefore the Lord blessed the Sabbath day and made it holy. (Exodus 20:8-11)

Then, there's *mental* rest. After I see 32 patients in the office, I'm sometimes mentally exhausted and just can't keep going without a change of focus. The brain needs downtime, just like the body. That's the beauty of restful worship. Both body and mind benefit tremendously.

So, how does one worship? The answer is very personal.

- Some worship best in **church.**
- Some worship during **Bible study**.
- Some talk directly to God in **prayer**.
- Some head out into **nature**, feeling close to God by observing His creation. Adam and Eve enjoyed this type of communion with their Creator.
- Some **serve others**. I remind myself of this in the hospital when I have to be on duty over the weekend and can't attend formal services.
- Some worship by the **mentoring of spiritual leaders**.
- Some worship by **thanking and praising God**.
- This **lesson you're reading** right now could be a form of worship.
- **Being obedient** to God's word is a beautiful act of worship.

The important message is to *come to God*. Ask Him to lead you into whatever type of worship fits your personality and needs the most. Then, when you're there, listen to His instruction and feel His love and closeness. Carefully examine how He's leading your life. You'll probably be surprised to see just how involved He is.

Our goal should be to remain in a constant state of worship so that, when the stones of life fly, we'll be calm and always have our eyes fixed on Jesus.

Look up 1 Thessalonians 5:17 and write down how often the Apostle Paul suggests we take part in the worship of prayer: _____

WRAPPING IT UP

Worship leads to rest and rest enables worship to be more effective. Both change our physiology in profound and sustainable ways. Chose your steps to a more perfect, restful worship and enjoy the benefits. Modern medicine can only do so much. An attitude of rest and worship can accomplish much.

LIVING IN COMMUNITY

As a group, think for a moment of how you worship. Then compile a poll.

How many:

Believe they worship primarily by Bible study and prayer? _____

Enjoy corporate worship? _____

Look for ways to serve others? _____

Find that nature suits them best? _____

Can't get enough praise and thanksgiving? _____

Look for mentors and small group studies? _____

Can you worship at work? _____

As a group, think of other ways we can worship God. Write them down here:

_____

_____

_____

_____

I suspect there will be much overlap. Remember, our goal is to live in constant worship and receive a constant flow of healing rest.

BEING MISSIONAL

Today, I want you to consider yourself to be on a mission to your neighbor. If you do not know your neighbor, go and introduce yourself. You can say something like: "Hi, I live next door and I just want to say hello. If you have an emergency and need help, don't hesitate to call on me. I'll do what I can." If you know them already, bring along a gift—like a loaf of delicious bread. Building relationships takes time. You have to begin somewhere. A simple act of kindness can change a life. It's also a form of worship.

COMMITMENT

Today, as you think about how you worship, commit to improving that all-important communion with God. Examine the ways you worship and ask God to lead you into even more meaningful methods and avenues.

Knowing what you know now, write down two simple action steps you can take to enhance your daily worship and your weekly worship. It may be as simple as turning your radio to a different station.

DAILY

  1. _____

  2. _____

WEEKLY

  1. _____

  2. _____

DAY 3

Changing the World

While we can't completely cover the complex subject of rest and worship in a mere week, the main point I want you to understand is that both change our chemistry. Today I'd like to turn our attention to Daniel.

As you may remember, God's chosen people kept turning away from God. So, at long last, God did what He usually does in times like that: He withdrew from their collective presence. The Bible describes it as "[letting] them go". This left the nation vulnerable and, sure enough, forces from outside their territory—outside of their Promised Land—rushed in and carried them away as captives. Daniel was one of those captives.

In time, because of his intellect and willingness to work hard—even for the nation that had dragged him away from his home—he rose in rank within the government and soon occupied a position of great authority. This made the non-captives under him angry, and they conspired to bring him down. How? They knew worship was important to Daniel. By requiring him to bow and worship someone other than the God of Heaven. They wrote a decree and then talked King Darius into signing it. Things were about to go from great to deadly for God's faithful captive.

Let's pick up the story to see what happened next.

> Now when Daniel knew that the writing was signed, he went home. And in his upper room, with his windows open toward Jerusalem, he knelt down on his knees three times that day, and prayed and gave thanks before his God, as was his custom since early days. Then these men assembled and found Daniel praying and making supplication before his God. And they went before the king, and spoke concerning the king's decree: "Have you not signed a decree that every man who petitions any god or man within thirty days, except you, O king, shall be cast into the den of lions? (Daniel 6:10-12)"

Most of us remember the rest of the story. Daniel continued to refuse to worship anyone but the God of Heaven and ended up right where his detractors wanted him: in the lions' den. After a rather uneasy night, he emerged uneaten. God had literally "shut the lions' mouth" (verse 22). Even with the thread of a violent death hanging over his head, Daniel would not compromise his worship.

In earlier days, Daniel was said to have been ten times smarter than the brightest in the kingdom. This was after he chose to eat pulse and water. I also believe that his wisdom was a result of the physiology of worship. For Daniel, communion with God through prayer was never compromised. He may not have had a church family with whom to worship. He didn't even own a Bible to read! But what he had—what he cherished most—was a dynamic and growing relationship with his Creator. Worship was a basic, irrefutable principle of life for him. He couldn't exist without it. As a result, his physiology was blessed.

"Worship" is a mere word that describes something special. It represents a relationship built on gratitude, awe, respect, obedience and love. But saying that, could worship also represent any activity that produces a specific measurable chemical and structural change in the brain? More to the point, can we learn to worship the wrong gods, the wrong philosophies, the wrong powers? We'll talk more about that later.

When it was time to cast Daniel into the lions' den, King Darius said, "Your God, whom you serve continually, He will deliver you" (Daniel 6:16). When the lions came, Daniel remained calm. His mind—like Christ's and Stephen's—had upshifted long before his date with the big cats. His brain didn't allow stress chemistry to dominate it.

His example of worship made a profound impact on King Darius. He declared in verse 25 through 27: "To all people, nations, and languages that dwell on earth: Peace be multiplied to you. I make a decree that in every dominion of my kingdom men must tremble and fear before the God of Daniel. For he is the living God. And steadfast forever; his kingdom is the one which shall not be destroyed, and his dominion shall endure to the end. He delivers and rescues, and He works signs and wonders in heaven and on earth, who has delivered Daniel from the power of the lions."

Amazing! Here's a ruler of the world proclaiming for the true God, all because of the worship of Daniel. Have you ever wondered if your worship is making a lasting impact on someone, somewhere? Keep in mind that God used Daniel's worship to change the world.

When lions are looming in your life, remember to gift yourself a daily and weekly rest from fear as you witness for your God. Remember to worship.

WRAPPING IT UP

Daniel didn't compromise. Worship was more important to him than his physical life. He knew that no matter happened, his God—the true God—would take care of him. He was assured of healing. Daniel didn't need to understand God's ways. He did not have the science of a whole food plant based diet. He did not have Dr. Newberg's studies on worship. He did not have studies on the human genome. He just trusted his Creator.

LIVING IN COMMUNITY

Today, think about the stories you've heard or read from the Bible concerning how people—from Adam and Eve to John the Revelator—worshiped the one true God. Write down four of the most common ways of worshiping here:

1. _____
2. _____
3. _____
4. _____

Which worship method most attracts you? _____

What can we learn from their worship?_____

How do other cultures in today's world worship?_____

How does worship vary even within your study group?_____

BEING MISSIONAL

Don't be afraid to witness to the King Dariuses of your world through worship. Think of two individuals in your life that might be influenced by seeing or knowing that you spend special time communing with God. You don't have to invite them to join you. Just say something like, "This week, during my special worship time, I'm going to be praying for you." Write their names below and begin praying for them right now.

1. _____
2. _____

COMMITMENT

Daniel was committed to prayer. It was the centerpiece of his worship. I want you to start discovering ways to talk to God regularly through prayer. Make it a priority to improve this part of your relationship with Him.

"I don't know how to pray," you may be saying. Well, relax. You're in good company. Christ's disciples weren't exactly sure either. They came to Him one day and said, "Teach us to pray." So, He did. Let's take a moment and sit at the feet of Jesus and allow Him to instruct us on how to talk to God in prayer.

> And when you pray, do not be like the hypocrites, for they love to pray standing in the synagogues and on the street corners to be seen by others. Truly I tell you, they have received their reward in full.

But when you pray, go into your room, close the door and pray to your Father, who is unseen. Then your Father, who sees what is done in secret, will reward you.

And when you pray, do not keep on babbling like pagans, for they think they will be heard because of their many words. Do not be like them, for your Father knows what you need before you ask him.

This, then, is how you should pray:

"Our Father in heaven, hallowed be your name, your kingdom come, your will be done, on earth as it is in heaven.

"Give us today our daily bread. And forgive us our debts, as we also have forgiven our debtors.

"And lead us not into temptation, but deliver us from the evil one. (Matthew 6:5-14)"

Short, simple, and to the point. You can add whatever else you feel like saying. God is eager to hear every word.

DAY 4

The Big Picture

Yesterday, I mentioned how words are mere representations of physiologic changes in the body. Here's an example. *Anxiety*. What exactly is anxiety? Can anxiety turn into a *phobia*? Is *post-traumatic stress* simply anxiety times a thousand? What about *fear*? I think you get the point. Words are often inadequate to explain the complexities of the mind and body. Yet, we need to use them to express ourselves.

Maybe someday we'll have access to the actual numbers and say: "This experience with Dana caused my epinephrine and cortisol to jump 50 points and inhibited my oxytocin count to a mere 12. Also, 30% of my anterior cingulate cortex became inactive and my amygdyla's response ramped up to 80. I also reactivated 14 circuits in the hippocampus!"

I make this point to demonstrate that we really know very little about God's creation. We're like a blindfolded man trying to describe an elephant by feel. That's why faith in His Word is an important aspect of worship. God can be trusted, even if we don't understand the reason why or know enough words to explain the physiology. The evidence supports trusting God.

Let's take a moment and memorize 2 Timothy 1:7 before we continue learning about worship:

| "For God has not given us a spirit of fear, but of power and of love and of sound mind."

Think about the time we spent learning about the brain. Remember the physiology of anxiety? It's a form of fear, especially *imagined* fear, which often comes from over-reacting, jumping to conclusions and taking things personally. These are learned behaviors that spring from inputs we've placed in our brains throughout a lifetime. They do absolutely nothing good for our ability to or enjoyment of worship. Fear and anxiety downshifts the brain, hurting cognitive ability and damaging our communion with our Creator.

God did not give us this physiology. According to the text we just memorized, He gave us power, love and a sound mind. This was our original DNA—the Heaven-ordained genetics implanted in our bodies. But, like everything else in this world, we've managed to mess up that original DNA and are now living in what best can be described as an "altered state."

Jeffery Dusek, PhD of Harvard Medical School, has studied how stress affects our DNA. Here's what he and his team of scientists discovered. Stress, which includes fear and anxiety, changes the expression of our genetic material. This means under stress, certain genes "switch on" or change. Since genes make amino acids and eventually the proteins that run the body, under stress, our bodies run differently.

But, as we revealed earlier in our study, stress has many causes. It might include not resting well, not drinking enough water, eating a poor diet, working too hard, keeping our brains on overload, poor relationships and even the uncertainty that comes from not worshipping the true God. The stress lists can be long! But these stresses aren't from God. He equipped us with the genetic encoding necessary to create love and a clear-thinking brain. He certainly didn't implant the stress chemistry that damages the body. That comes when we alter our minds and bodies through fear and anxiety.

Listen to this: Dr. Dusek has found 2209 genes associated with chronic medical problems that are expressed differently under stress. These include genes that effect aging, the immune system, inflammation and even physical thinning of the brain. I don't know about you, but I don't want my brain any thinner than it already is!

These genes also contribute to oxidative stress, which is harmful to many bodily systems including the cardiovascular. Yes, stress changes our DNA and our very brain. Research has shown how stress causes the telomeres on our DNA to shorten. The telomeres help keep the DNA functioning optimally. We want longer and not shorter telomeres. Less stress means the DNA is better equipped to repair and remain functioning at optimal levels.

Why do I bring this up? As we learn about worship today—and for the rest of our lives—we'll discover more and more evidence that God's plan is best for us. I'm reminded of 1 John 4:18 where we're told "Love casts out all fear." That's right. God has given us the treatment for stress, which alters DNA. And that treatment is *love*.

As with everything else, love is just a word representing chemical changes. So, we can use science-speak to paraphrase that verse to read, "The chemical change called 'love' can reverse the chemical change called 'fear.'" Isn't that good to know! What a wonderful God we worship!

We've discovered that the opposite of love (others-focused) is selfishness (self-focused). Selfishness embodies the "me first" mentality. It's the "live for the moment" response that triggers the lower functions of the brain. That's downshifting. The lower parts of the brain, if you recall, are what we share with reptiles and mammals. The more these circuits are activated the more the higher parts, with their executive functions, are diminished. And herein lies a problem. Selfishness hinders our ability to worship. Why? Love turns down the stress chemistry and upshifts the brain. It activates the anterior cingulate cortex to develop caring, abstract thought, increase our understanding of metaphors and ultimately making it possible to better communicate (worship) with God.

Then an amazing thing happens. Worship—connecting with God—strengthens our ability and desire to love. A circle is formed. New neural pathways are developed. And before long, our very DNA adjusts to the new reality that's now driving our lives. We are moving toward a chemistry of rest and not stress. The DNA is improved, longer telomeres, but probably much more is going on that we still have not discovered.

I John 4:8 reads, "Whoever does not love does not know God, because God is love." There you have it.

- To cast out fear and get our physiology heading in the right direction requires turning on love and turning off selfishness.

- It requires an upshifting of the brain that expresses the DNA that generates the good chemistry we were designed to enjoy.

- In order to know God, we have to worship Him.

- The more we worship Him, the more we love Him whom turns off our fear.

- Worship thus can be described as a treatment.

This is so important to understand! I want you to store this information deep in your hippocampus forever.

I believe we've improved our brain during our studies together. Hopefully, it's a transformation that you'll continue to address long after our time together has ended. Worship gives us the power to change and the power to be unique when everyone else is heading down a different path.

WRAPPING IT UP

The stress of a world living contrary to the original plan puts stress on everyone's body. We now have the technology necessary to begin to understand what's happening to us on the molecular level. But, there's so much more to learn. I have a feeling that the knowledge we accrue will highlight even more truths hidden in the Bible. As we adopt these truths, our physiology will continue to improve as well.

One thing we can know right now: A powerful Biblical Prescription for stress is rest and worship. These gifts from God reinvigorate our physiology and create improvement of gene expression, which brings positive structural and chemical changes in the brain.

LIVING IN COMMUNITY

Yesterday, I asked you to talk within your group about how they worship. I hope a few texts, emails, or phone calls were exchanged.

You've probably heard of Dr. Gary Chapman's book "Understanding the Five Love Languages" (Northfield Publishing, 1995). As a review, they are:

1. Gifts

2. Quality Time

3. Words of Affirmation

4. Acts of Service

5. Physical Touch

Today, discuss within your group what love language works best for each member. Then talk about whether there's a connection between their love language and how they worship. (There usually is).

Then discuss ways that Jesus fulfilled each and every language. Write your answers here:

1. Gifts _____

2. Quality Time _____

3. Words of Affirmation_____

4. Acts of Service _____

5. Physical Touch _____

BEING MISSIONAL

Pick someone that you know. Find a way to lower his or her stress. When you do this, you're moving that person in the direction of love and worship. You are being a flesh-and-blood Biblical Prescription to the world. Be creative. If you can't think of any way in particular, simply smile or deliver a hearty hug. I want you to document the results here:

Person 1   Name: _____

Here's how I lowered his/her stress: _____

Results: _____

Person 2   Name: _____

Here's how I lowered his/her stress: _____

Results: _____

By the way, if you want to practice on a pet, that would be fine.

When you do this assignment, you're being a healer—a treatment for the world. Jesus met needs everywhere He went. He loved and didn't judge. By doing so, He moved people one step closer to a relationship with His Father. This is our mission today.

COMMITMENT

Take 30 minutes today to be alone. Review the "Big Picture" and answer these questions:

- What are you here to accomplish? _____
- How can you lower the stress of yourself, your family and the world? _____

If you're not sure where to start, ask God to show you His will for your life. Don't expect everything at once.

DAY 5

Definitions of a Word

By now, I hope we're all beginning to understand how vital worship is to our health. As we've pointed out, it's part of the fabric of life; a universal truth. Even if we don't believe in the law of gravity, if we jump off a building there will be consequences. If we don't believe in worship and if we fail to do it, there will be physiologic consequences.

Keep in mind that those consequences aren't a punishment from God. They're simply what happen when a universal truth is ignored. For example, consider what happens when you don't consider gravity.

Worship is a word with a deep meaning. In Dr. Newberg's research we explored earlier, those who worshiped had a changed physiology. It's clear to me that our goal is to worship the true God.

Today I'd like to address these questions:

- What is worship?
- How do we know when we're worshiping?
- Is worship the same for everyone?

A dictionary definition of worship is "the reverent love and devotion accorded to a deity, an idol, or sacred object." Here are some other definitions/descriptions:

Southern pastor **Louie Giglio** describes worship as "our response both personal and corporate, to God for who

He is and what He has done; expressed in and by the things we say and the way we live."

Christian author **Harold Best** insists "worship is the sign that in giving myself completely to someone or something else, I want to be mastered by it."

Theologian **David Peterson** says, "Worship of the living and true God is essentially an engagement with Him on the terms He proposes and in the way He alone makes possible."

Archbishop **William Temple** writes: "To worship is to quicken the conscious to the holiness of God, to feed the mind with the wonderful truth of God, to purge the imagination in the beauty of God, to open the heart to the love of God, to devote the will to the purpose of God."

Research professor **D. A. Carson** suggests: "To worship God in spirit and truth, worship God by means of Christ."

Worship.com's founder **Josh Riley** shares that worship is "everything we think, everything we say, and everything we do, revealing that which we treasure and value most in life."

Pastor **Mark Driscoll** tells his congregation that worship is "living our life individually and corporately as continued living sacrifices to the glory of a person or thing."

Others describe worship as a "friendship" and "intimacy with God." We saw in Enoch a "walk with God." In Daniel we saw continued communication and obedience to God.

These are all words trying to describe something that's not a word. Perhaps one scientific definition could be "the physiologic state of the body in which the anterior cingulate cortex grows and forms new neural pathways with increased production of oxytocin, endorphins, GABA, and dopamine while decreasing the stress physiology of the body as the human mind puts the interests of others above its own in a continued relationship with the true God."

As we can see, there are many ways to worship God. One of the ways I worship best is in nature. A walk in the forest or a stroll along a beach in beautiful weather represents the most meaningful worship for me. Just as Stephen and Daniel found rest and ultimately strength in worship, as you commune with God, this will change you and give rest that counteracts stress physiology. What a wonderful gift to open!

Think again about your worship in the light of the above definitions. Checkmark those types of worship that appeal to you most:

❏   Attending church

❏   Reading God's Word

❏   Spending time in prayer

- ❏ Serving others

- ❏ Experiencing creation in nature

- ❏ Caring for God's gifts to you including your body, children, and relationships

- ❏ Taking part in Bible studies like this one

- ❏ Listening to mentors (pastors, teachers, friends)

- ❏ Offering thanks and praise to God

- ❏ My own special worship not listed here is _____

I suspect that your worship, like mine, contains elements of many. But I'm sure you have favorites.

Let's do a little exercise. Here's that list again, but this time answer "Why" to each item. Why do I enjoy worshiping in this manner?

- ❏ Attending church: _____

- ❏ Reading God's Word: _____

- ❏ Spending time in prayer: _____

- ❏ Serving others: _____

- ❏ Experiencing creation in nature: _____

- ❏ Caring for God's gifts to you including your body, children, and relationships:

  _____

- ❏ Taking part in Bible studies like this one: _____

- ❏ Listening to mentors: _____

- ❏ Offering thanks and praise to God: _____

- ❏ My own special worship: _____

In whatever way we choose, if we spend time with our Heavenly Father, *we will be changed*. As we worship the true God, our physiology will be transformed.

WRAPPING IT UP

One of the goals with this series of lessons is to maximize your worship through better health, less stress, and a clearer communication with the Creator. To that we can add:

- Taking the necessary time out of our busy schedule to share what we've learned.

- To encourage those around us.

- To love one another as God has loved us.

Worship means many things and can even be described by the physiologic changes it produces in the brain.

LIVING IN COMMUNITY

In your group, discuss the way people worshiped before the Bible, as we know it was compiled and translated into English. This took place in 1611 with the commissioning of the King James Bible. Answer the following questions:

- Do you think it's easier to worship in our modernized world? _____
- Why do you think that? _____
- If you were born around the time of Christ, how would you have been worshipping?

  _____

- How about in the time of Moses?_____
- How did Adam and Eve worship? _____

Our God is the same. Universal truths are constant. Consider this text and write down how this announcement impacts your worship.

For I the Lord do not change. (Malachi 3:6)

_____

_____

BEING MISSIONAL

Write a letter to someone today. It may be to a friend, family member, neighbor, or spouse. In this letter, find a way to spread the idea that worship changes the body. You could always keep a copy of your letter on file for future use when God impresses you to send it to someone who is searching.

COMMITMENT

I hope you have the ability go outside today. Find something in nature and observe. This might be a flower or an insect or even cloud gazing. Write down your observations below.

_____

_____

Yes. This is worship!

DAY 6

A New Heart

One day I noticed my son on his cell phone. "Are you texting God?" I asked. He gave me a puzzled look and then frowned. "You can't text God," he said. "Are you sure?" I pressed.

Don't ever underestimate the God of the universe. If He can speak a solar system into existence and form a living human from a little pile mud, He's probably more than capable of sending and receiving text messages on a smart phone.

Yesterday, we learned that worship is a word that could mean different things to different people. Our relationship with God helps determine it's meaning to us. Since there are many ways to worship God, we must never underestimate His willingness and response whenever *and however* we communicate with Him through heart-felt worship. Just ask David.

Good ol' David was a man who, after the incident with Bathsheba, knew his mind was not making good decisions. He'd let his carnal nature eclipse his divine nature in a rather profound way. Looking back over his life—and the horrendous things he'd done—he made an interesting request of God.

Using your Bible, fill in the blanks of this text to discover King David's strange request.

Psalm 51:19: "_____ in me a _____ _____, O God; and _____ a right _____ within me."

David knew where to go to for healing and he was not too proud to ask for it. When he felt a need, what did he do? He worshiped God. Thanking and praising the Lord in all things is a beautiful way to commune with the Creator.

Consider these beautiful words of worship written by a man who made terrible mistakes, but who chose worship over guilt and praise over self-condemnation. Circle the action verbs that form the foundation of his worship. The first word is "Make."

> Make a joyful noise to the Lord, all the earth! Serve the Lord with gladness! Come into his presence with singing! Know that the Lord, he is God! It is he who made us, and we are his; we are his people, and the sheep of his pasture. Enter his gates with thanksgiving, and his courts with praise! Give thanks to him; bless his name! For the Lord is good; his steadfast love endures forever, and his faithfulness to all generations. (Psalm 100:1-5)

Do we know how, in this modern era, to be thankful? Researchers have shown that it's virtually impossible to be truly thankful and fearful at the same time. Why? Because thankfulness and praise upshift the brain and improve cognitive ability. A thankful heart is a happy heart with endorphins being released left and right. Fear doesn't stand a chance in that chemical stew of joy. When in this upshifted frame of mind, we can also watch our DNA adjust itself to our new reality of happiness. Wow.

Let's do a little exercise to get that transformation under way. Read the following texts and then write down an area of your life that will benefit by your following that text's advice or message. This is worship at its most fundamental and powerful level: God's Word versus our struggles.

Psalm 27:14: Wait for the Lord; be strong and take heart and wait on the Lord.

_____

2 Kings 6:16: "Don't be afraid," the prophet answered. "Those who are with us are more than those who are with them."

_____

Psalm 46:1, 2: God is our refuge and strength, an ever-present help in trouble. Therefore will not we fear, though the earth give way and the mountains fall into the heart of the sea.

_____

Psalm 37:24: Though he stumble, he will not fall, for the Lord upholds him with his hand.

_____

Proverbs 1:33: But whoever listens to me will live in safety and be at ease, without fear of harm.

_____

Isaiah 30:21: Whether you turn to the right or to the left, your ears will hear a voice behind you, saying, "This is the way; walk in it."

_____

Psalm 73:26: My flesh and my heart may fail, but God is the strength of my heart and my portion forever.

_____

Psalm 42:11: Why, my soul, are you downcast? Why so disturbed within me? Put your hope in God for I will yet praise him, my Savior and my God.

_____

Now place a star beside the text that means the most to you. Commit it to memory right now! Consider it your most powerful upshift verse.

Let's review for a moment. During this Bible study course, we've studied how:

- Our physical lives and spiritual lives are intertwined.

- Stress contributes to illness.

- Rest through worship heals mind and body by changing our entire chemistry and physiology.

- Physical water bathes every cell while "Living Water" cleanses the soul.

- Light is necessary for Vitamin D activation, cellular function, and much more while the "Light of Truth" is necessary for faith formation and successful life function.

- Walking for health can remind us to walk with God.

- Eating nutritious food reverses diseases and speeds healing while partaking of "the Bread of Life" reverses the destructive direction of our life and speeds the healing of our spirit.

- Developing—with God's help—a healthy mind allows God to create a new mind in us and change us from the inside out.

We now have the technology necessary to prove, again and again, what God has promised. I think that's astonishing! It's now time to thank and praise God for His endless love; love that casts out all fear. Jesus said that the very hairs of our head are numbered (Matthew 10:30). But, as we've discovered, that's just the tip of the iceberg for what God knows about us. He truly loves us from the inside out. Take a moment right now and personally—or as a group—bow your head and just think about the matchless, wonderful love of the Creator.

WRAPPING IT UP

David had problems. He knew where to go for the solution. He needed a new heart, a new mind. I, like David, need a new heart. My genetics are stressed out. If I treat my symptoms and not the cause, I will not have healing. But I know where to go for answers. And so do you.

LIVING IN COMMUNITY

Have your group make a list of seven things for which they are most thankful. Record them here:

1. _____

2. _____

3. _____

4. _____

5. _____

6. _____

7. _____

It's important to finish this list. Thankfulness, like laughter, is contagious.

BEING MISSIONAL

Make it a point to express thanks to everyone with whom you come in contact today. Simply remember an act of kindness or a bit of encouragement or inspiration that someone offered in the past and tell him/her how much you appreciate them. Start with the Creator and make a list below of those you plan to thank today. I'm hopeful there will be more than three. I appreciate each one of you who are taking this course and making changes for life.

1. Jesus

2. _____

3. _____

4. _____

COMMITMENT

Make a commitment to think back on your life and make a list of how God has led you in the past even when you hadn't asked Him to. This may have been times when you were not worshiping or listening for His voice. Remember, God doesn't do what He does because we love Him. He does what He does because He loves us. Jot down the list below.

_____

_____

_____

DAY 7

Our Generous God

When we "turn our eyes upon Jesus" as the song says, we're worshiping Him. But, we're also doing something else: we're getting healing. The same Jesus we worship has authority over illness. He's a treatment for our diseases. We can ask Him to heal us from the inside out and He will—in His way and in His time.

Then, when we feed the hungry, help the sick, clothe those without protection, and find ways to love another soul, we're simply returning the favor. In essence, we're taking care of Jesus! "Whatever you did for one of the least of these brothers and sisters of mine, you did for me," He told His disciples in Matthew 25:40. This is love in action. This brand of love offers many positive side effects. It casts out fear, changes our chemistry for the good, and redirects us back toward our original design.

Our goal should not be to simply attend church or read our Bibles more. No, our goal is to *live* in worship—to have it be the central theme of life. This will optimize health because, as we've learned during these lessons, there's a firm link between the physical and spiritual aspects of our being. Good physical health improves our spiritual health. Then that growing and dynamic spiritual health improves our physical health. What a powerful and uplifting cycle! Today's technology offers ample evidence to prove that connection over and over again.

Besides our daily need for rest, please don't forget that all-important Sabbath rest. It's an opportunity to worship while gaining the physical, mental, and spiritual rest we need to reverse damaging stress physiology.

Solomon, the wisest man in the world, wrote in Proverbs 3:6, "In all your ways acknowledge Him, and He shall direct your paths."

Memorize this text. This is another promise. When we turn to God for answers to the questions of life, He has promised to direct our paths. This has been our goal during these lessons to worship/acknowledge God and He would direct our paths, our steps. In health this might be an understanding of why we are sick, steps to improve our water intake or going outside and moving. As we acknowledge and worship Him today, tomorrow, and over a lifetime, God will direct our paths. I hope right now you know that this is happening in your life.

As we are nearing the end of this study, I hope you will continue to think about and process all that we've learned. Today, if the Holy Spirit is tugging at your heart, why not accept God's gift of salvation? If you've already accepted this gift, commit yourself to growing your relationship with the Creator like never before. I thank God for the time we've shared and look forward to meeting each one of you someday.

If need be, take some time and repeat this study down the road. Use this study as a tool to help spread the gospel. Invite a few friends who you think and lead a group. We are here to help. If you have questions or would like special prayer, don't hesitate to contact me at one of our websites: biblicalprescriptionsforlife.com or heartwiseministries.org. Just know that our entire Heartwise team will be praying for you. And remember:

If any of you lacks wisdom, let him ask God, who gives generously to all without reproach, and it will be given him. (James 1:5)

Continue in the rest God gives as you worship Him today, tomorrow and for eternity.